Edible and Medicinal Plants of the Rocky Mountains

A Beginner's Guide to Medicinal Wild Plants of the Rockies

Christopher O. Daniel

Contents

INTRODUCTION

A Guide to Edible and Medicinal Plants of the Rockies" explores the diverse array of plant life that adorns this awe-inspiring region and potentially provides healing and sustenance.

You will be transported into the untamed splendor of the Rockies as you peruse the contents of this guide. In this region, every plant serves as a poetic representation of the intricate interplay between nature and humanity, as well as adaptation and resilience. This book acts as a companion as you explore secluded valleys and windswept alpine meadows, revealing the secrets of the diverse plant life that flourishes in this one-of-a-kind ecosystem.

Our objective is to establish a connection between keen explorers and the abundant resources bestowed upon us by nature. This comprehensive and user-friendly manual assists individuals of all skill levels—from seasoned foragers to inquisitive hikers to those in search of a more profound understanding of the environment—in locating, gathering, and making use of the edible and medicinal plants that inhabit the Rocky Mountains.

The following chapters will explore the folklore and traditional applications of these organisms, disclosing their medicinal properties, nutritional value, and culinary uses. By means of succinct explanations, evocative visuals, and pragmatic observations, this book will furnish you with the understanding and assurance necessary to initiate your own foraging expeditions in the Rocky Mountains, thereby establishing a symbiotic connection with the environment and its botanical marvels.

Prepare yourself for an intellectually stimulating expedition as we traverse the Rockies—a voyage that delves beneath the aesthetic allure of the terrain and unveils an extraordinary realm of medicinal and edible plants that have subtly flourished for millennia, awaiting our acknowledgment of their value and acceptance of the abundant natural resources that encompass us.

CHAPTER ONE

BENEFITS OF NATURAL HERBAL REMEDIES

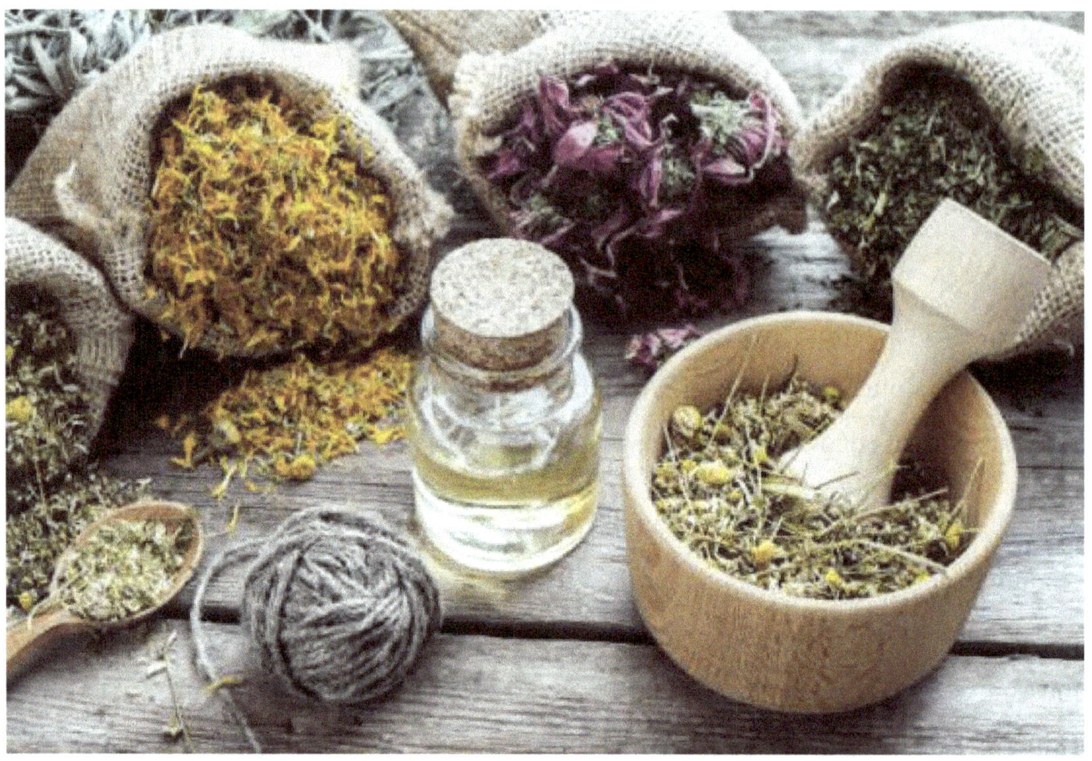

Historically acknowledged and substantiated by contemporary research, natural herbal remedies derived from plants indigenous to Canada present an array of prospective advantages.

Despite the potential benefits of herbal remedies, it is crucial to exercise caution and seek appropriate guidance when utilizing them. Listed below are some potential benefits of herbal remedies derived from flora native to the Canada:

- **Traditional Healing Methods**

Numerous herbal remedies have been used in traditional medicinal practices for centuries. Historical plant uses and indigenous knowledge have been transmitted across generations, serving as the foundation for herbal medication.

- **Assistance for Frequent Illnesses**

It is believed that numerous herbs can provide alleviation from common ailments, including coughs, colds, digestive issues, and headaches. Peppermint and chamomile, for instance, are recognized for their digestive properties, whereas elderberry is frequently applied topically to alleviate the symptoms of the common cold.

- **Antimicrobial Characteristics**

Certain herbs, such as sage and thyme, are renowned in the Canada for their antimicrobial attributes. Historically, thyme has been employed as a therapeutic intervention for respiratory infections.

- **Effects Anti-Inflammatory**

Despite the fact that turmeric and ginger are not indigenous to the Canada, their anti-inflammatory properties make them commonplace. Traditional use of meadowsweet, a plant native to the Canada, has included analgesic and potentially anti-inflammatory properties.

- **Management of Anxiety and Stress**

Lavender and lemon balm are frequent examples of herbs utilized for their stress-relieving and soothing attributes. These botanicals could potentially facilitate the process of relaxation and bolster mental health.

- **Enhancement of sleep quality**

Native to the Canada, Valerian root has historically been used as a sleep aid. It could possibly facilitate relaxation and enhance the quality of sleep.

- **Packed with nutrients**

Certain edible botanicals and plants contain an abundance of antioxidants, vitamins, and minerals. For example, nettles are rich in iron, vitamins A and C, and various minerals.

- **Regarding skin care**

Herbal remedies that target conditions such as eczema and dermatitis frequently contain calendula and chamomile, which are renowned for their soothing attributes.

- **Gentle and Holistic Approach:**

Herbal remedies are often regarded as a more compassionate and holistic approach to health, placing emphasis on the comprehensive well-being of the user.

When considering herbal remedies, it is critical to exercise prudence, particularly if one has pre-existing medical conditions or is currently taking medications.

It is advisable to seek guidance from a certified healthcare practitioner or herbalist prior to integrating herbal remedies into one's daily healthcare regimen. It is also necessary to adhere to ethical and sustainable harvesting methods in order to safeguard plant populations.

CHAPTER TWO

MULLEIN

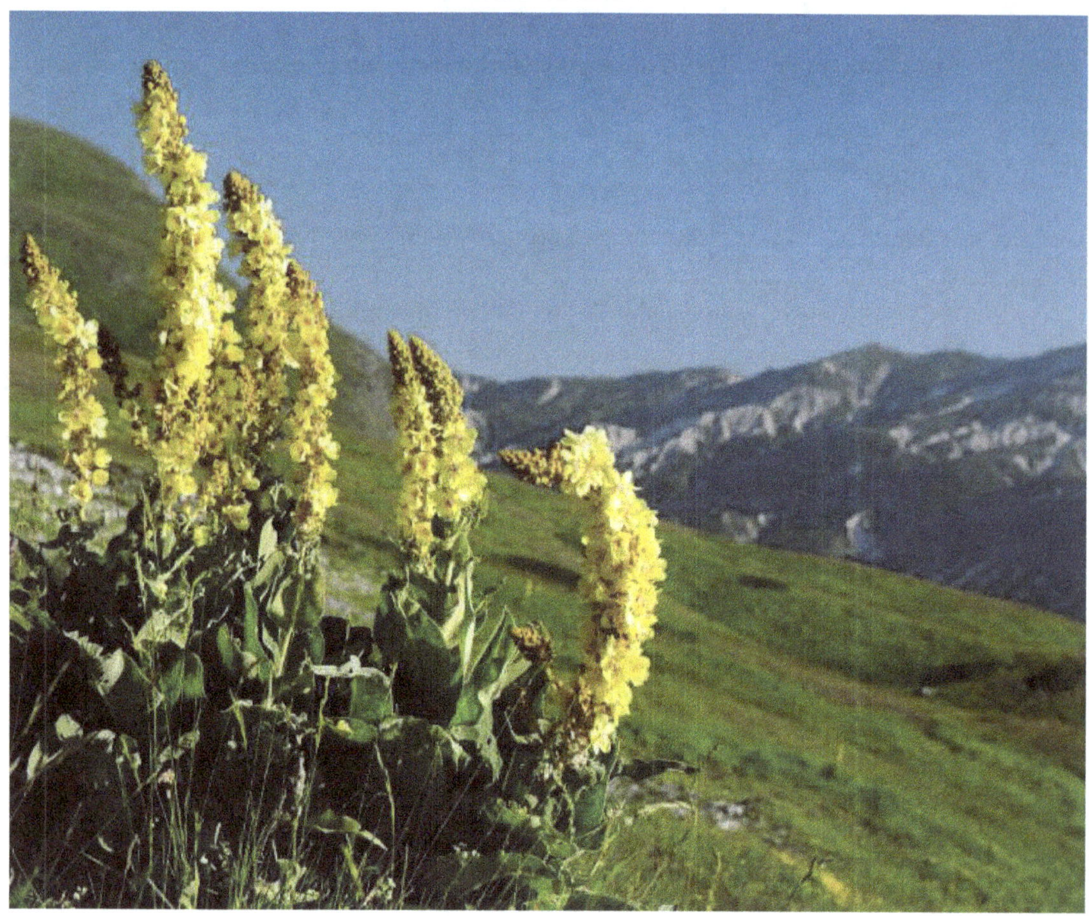

A species of mullein native to Europe, northern Africa, and Asia, Verbascum thapsus, was introduced to the Americas and Australia. It is also known as the great mullein, greater mullein, or common mullein.

This bushy biennial can attain a maximum height of 2 meters. Dense clusters of small, yellow flowers adorn a tall stem that originates from a sizable rosette of foliage.

It may emerge shortly after the ground receives light from long-lasting seeds that persist in the soil seed bank in well-lit, disturbed soils, although it can grow in a wide variety of habitats. It is a prevalent weed that proliferates by producing seeds and has become invasive in temperate regions of the world.

This species poses a negligible threat to the majority of agricultural commodities due to its lack of competitiveness, intolerance for shade from other plants, and inability to withstand tilling. A number of the insects that inhabit it are also potentially hazardous to other flora.

Permanently eradicating populations is more challenging than manually removing members of an individual.

While this plant is frequently employed in traditional medicine, no FDA-approved pharmaceuticals are derived from it. It has been incorporated into torches and dyes.

Identification

Mullein has a tall, erect stem in its second year that has the potential to grow very high. This wild edible has yellow flowers atop the plant and soft foliage, giving it a distinctive appearance.

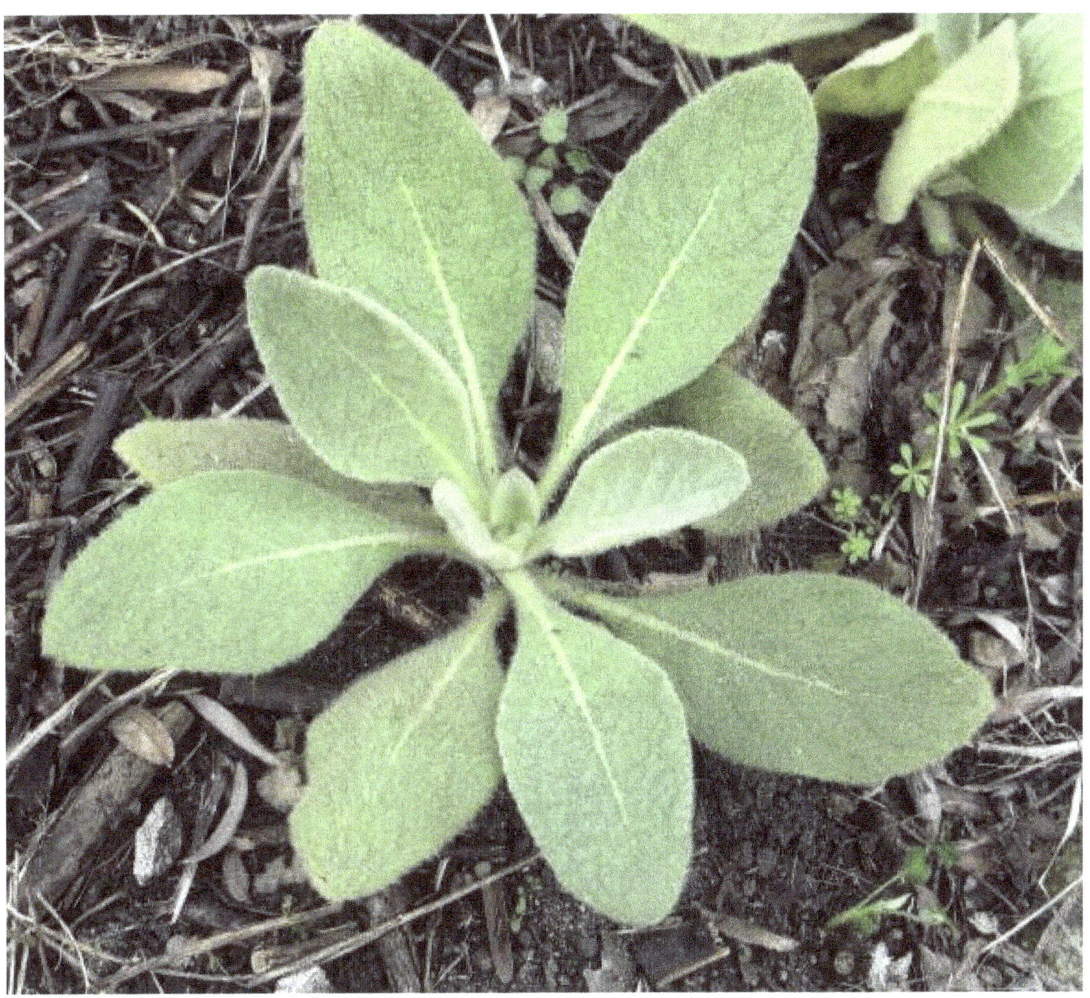

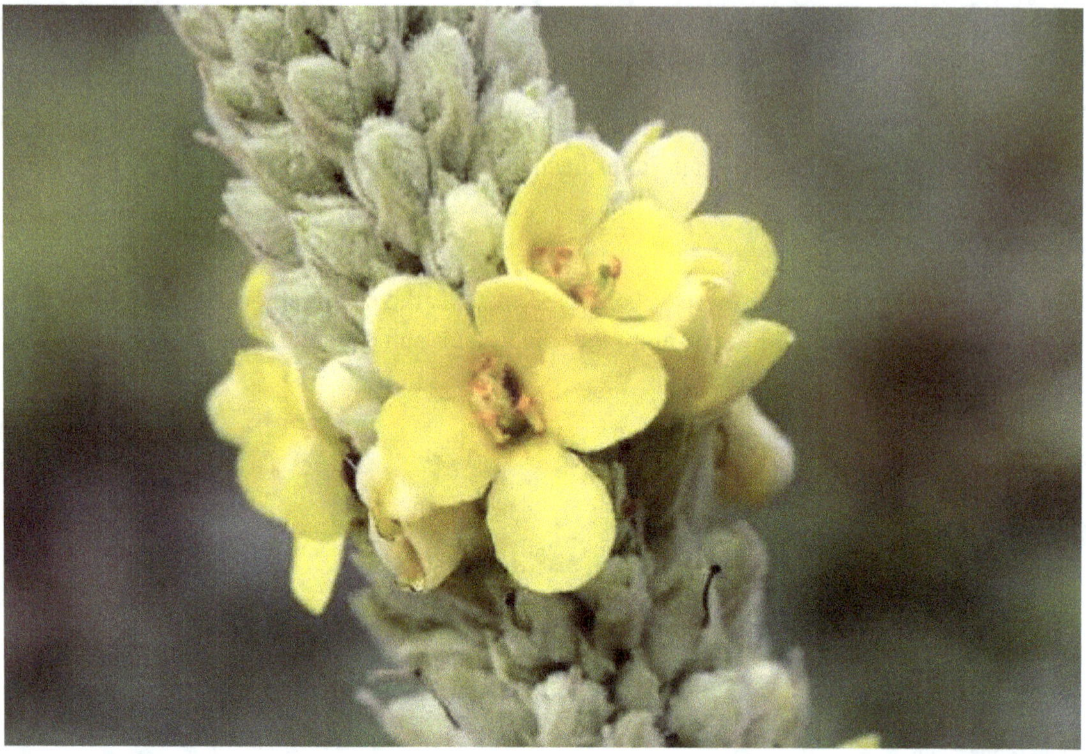

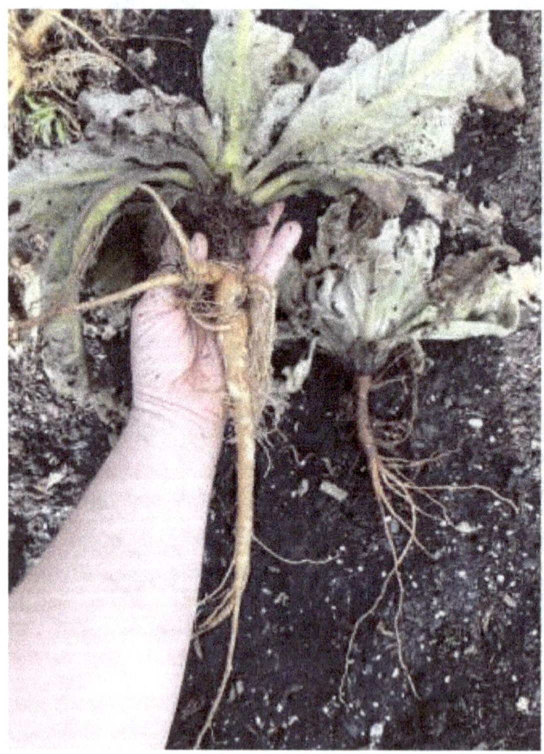 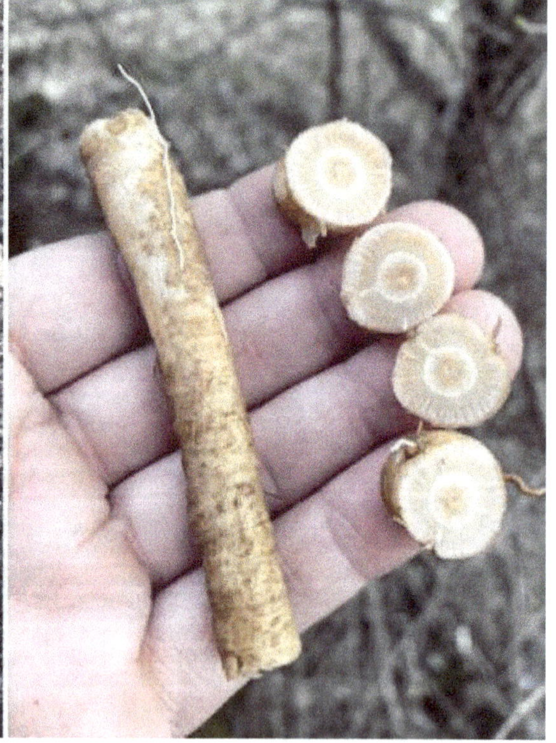

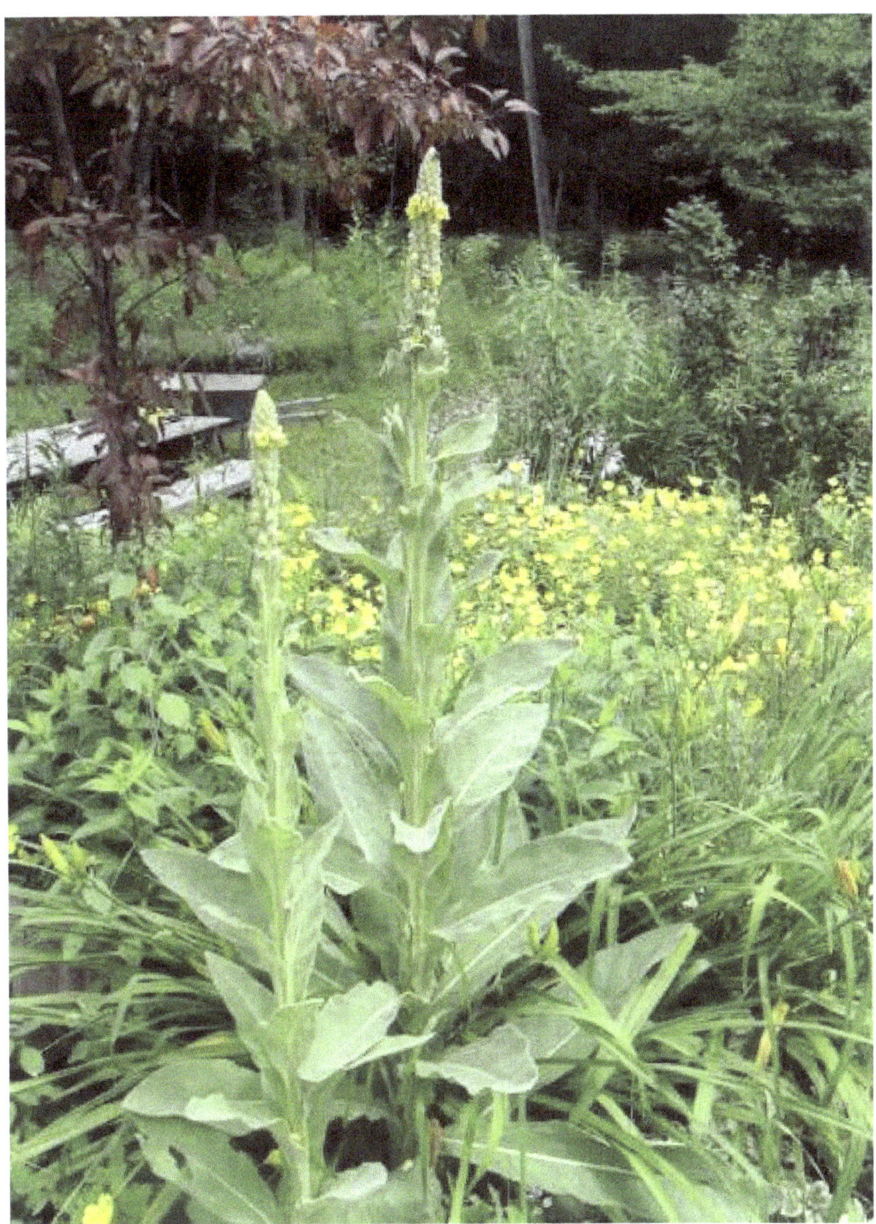

- **Flowers**

The mullein plant's central stem culminates in a compact spike of pale yellow flowers, which typically range in length from 5 to 60 cm (equivalent to 2" to 2').

Each flower has five pallid petals, five hairy green sepals, five stamens, and a pistil; it measures about 2 cm (½") in diameter. The two lower filaments are devoid of hairs, whereas the three upper stamens are adorned with yellow or white hairs.

The blooming period typically lasts for approximately six weeks and occurs during the summer. A limited number of blossoms are present during any given period. Every individual flower is substituted with a seed capsule comprising two cells, wherein each cell harbors an abundance of minuscule seeds.

- **Leaves**

The first year of mullein development results in the formation of a basal rosette comprised of 50 cm-long, velvety-like, long elliptical leaves in a shade of gray-green. In the second year, a robust, upright floral stalk emerges before the basal leaves.

- **Roots**

Each Mullein plant grows a deep tap root and system of fibrous roots allowing it to overwinter and withstand drought.

- **Seeds**

After flowering, Mullein produces small ¼-inch ovoid seed capsules. These capsules split open and release large numbers of tiny, ridged, brown seeds less than 0.04 inches in length. These seeds are toxic.

- **Height**

Mullein can reach heights of just over 2 meters.

- **Edible parts**

Flowers and foliage. While the leaves and flowers are edible, it is generally more enjoyable to consume a cup of tea prepared from these components. Flowers and leaves may be incorporated into a salad.

- **Other Name**

Cowboy toilet paper

- **Flavor**

Similar to peppermint in flavor, mullein is a mildly sweet wellness beverage that can be easily consumed to treat coughs, colds, bronchitis, and other ailments. For good reason, mullein is one of our most popular herbal teas.

Season

Preferably in the late spring or early summer

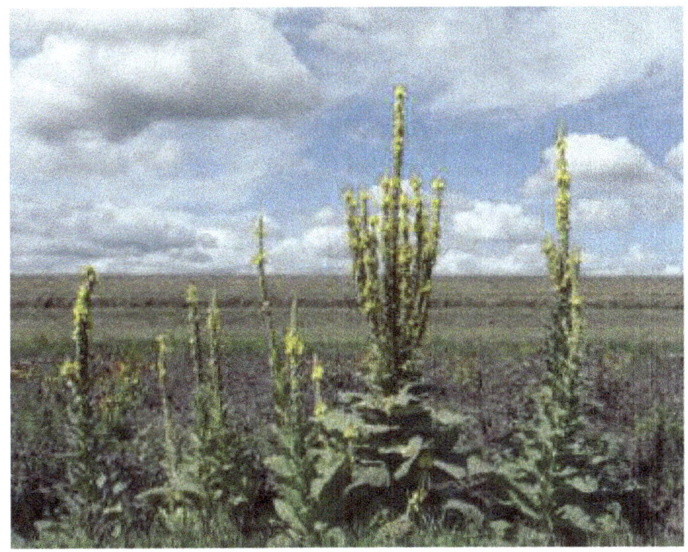

Mullein is commonly observed flourishing in arid, sunlit regions such as open fields, wastelands, disturbed areas, and railway embankments.

Medicinal Benefits

Mullein is a fundamental herb in a number of traditional customs. Mullein was first mentioned in history two millennia ago, when the renowned Greek physician Dioscorides prescribed it for pulmonary diseases. Typically, the leaves were smoked for this purpose.

Over the years, oil infused with Mullein flowers has been utilized for the treatment of a variety of external conditions, including earaches, frostbite, eczema, warts, and sores. Various preparations have been employed for the treatment of ailments such as croup, colds, flu, and ulcers.

Traditional Austrian medicine employed Mullien for external applications such as compresses, ointments, and baths, as well as internally as a tea. Concerns pertaining to the epidermis, gastrointestinal tract, lungs, veins, and muscles were addressed with these preparations.

After colonists introduced Mullein to North America, Native Americans quickly adapted it. The practice of smoking the leaves and powdered roots, as well as preparing tea, was maintained. Some groups, including the Zuni, discovered additional applications. The Zuni utilized pulverized root poultices as a remedy for skin infections, ulcers, and rashes. In addition, an infusion was utilized to treat the athlete's foot.

In the Makaland region of Pakistan, certain communities employ Mullein as an additional vermicide. A study from 2012 provided support for this usage. An efficacy assessment of Mullein extract was conducted by researchers on roundworms and tapeworms.

Modern research has, to some extent, supported the use of mullein by herbalists to treat various lung diseases and infections. Mullein possesses antiseptic properties and is effective against pneumonia, MRSA, and E. coli bacteria, according to a 2002 study.

In spite of the fact that folk herbalists assert that a tincture of mullein root is particularly effective for back discomfort, scientific research has yet to validate this claim.

Ways to Use Mullein

Mullein is non-palatable as an untamed herb, despite the fact that it is edible and can be consumed in a survival situation. Mullein is more suitable for use in medicinal formulations.

The flowers of the Mullein plant can be used to make an infused oil. Mullein flowers, foliage, and roots can be incorporated into ointments, poultices, and baths. They can be employed to formulate beverages, infusions, and tinctures for internal consumption. Additionally, desiccated and smoked mullein leaves and roots can be used for medicinal purposes.

Additionally, mullein flowers can be preserved in sugar to produce mullein syrup, in addition to being frequently infused into oil. As the sugar extracts the moisture from the blossoms, the entire mixture transforms into a viscous syrup that provides sore throat relief.

Various cultures throughout history, including the Romans and Native American tribes, have used dried Mullein stems to make torches or candles. In order to produce one, the desiccated stem must be dipped in wax multiple times until a thick layer forms. These torches were utilized for ritual or survival purposes.

Native Americans obtained additional sustenance from this intriguing plant. Mullein seeds comprise rotenone, a chemical compound that induces paralysis in fish. Native Americans ground the seeds and used them to catch fish.

Mullein has been cultivated for ornamental purposes as well. There are numerous ornamental cultivars that feature more flamboyant flowers compared to the majority of their natural counterparts.

How to Grow

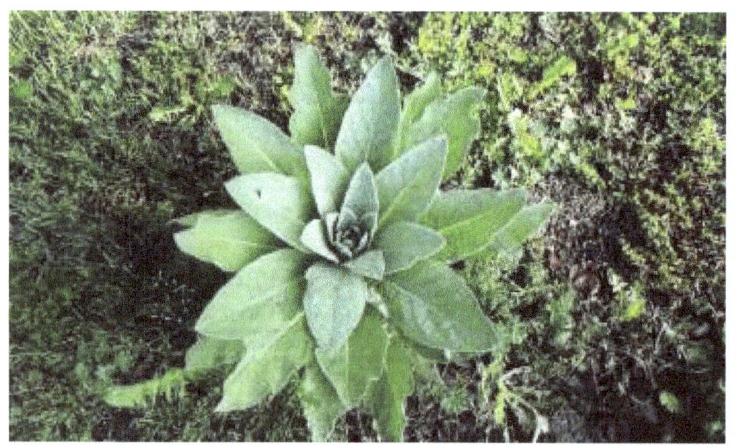

Mullein plants can attain a maximum height of 6 feet, creating a distinctive setting. Its leaves can attain a maximum width of 2 feet and can protrude significantly within a garden plot.

- **Appropriate soil for Mullein**

The fact that mullein develops along roadside areas suggests that this plant does not place a high value on soil quality. Although it can thrive in a wide range of soil types, mullein prefers well-draining, calcareous soil. The optimal conditions for plant development are arid, slightly alkaline soil.

- ### The Right Location for Growing Mullein

Above all else, keep in mind that Mullein requires ample space to develop. Given that this plant has the potential to attain a maximum height of 10 feet, it is imperative that you choose a location devoid of any compromised space. Certain novel cultivars attain a maximum height of 5 feet.

Other than space, mullein prefers warm, arid environments with direct sunlight. This herb thrives in close proximity to structures or large trees, which will provide wind protection. Bear in mind that these are lofty plants, which means that strong winds could potentially harm them.

- ### Starting Mullein from Seeds

Mullein is capable of being propagated via seed or cuttings. Gather seeds from vegetation in the immediate moment they emerge. Additionally, one may acquire seedlings.

Mullein seedlings should be sown indoors during the early spring. Ensure that the seedlings are started indoors six to eight weeks prior to the last snowfall of the spring.

Prior to thoroughly saturating the potting soil, distribute seeds on its surface. Expect two weeks for mullein seeds to germinate; therefore, exercise patience. The appearance of the seedlings requires some time. In late spring, you may also distribute the seeds directly into the garden. This may require additional time, so ensure you have a sufficient growing season to accomplish it.

After the seedlings have emerged, reduce them. Once the plants develop their true foliage, you may transplant them to a larger container or the ground as they mature.

- ### Mullein's Planting in the Garden

The spacing between greater plants varies by variety but generally requires a distance of 3 feet. Plant shorter varieties at a distance of 12 to 14 inches apart

How to Care for Mullein

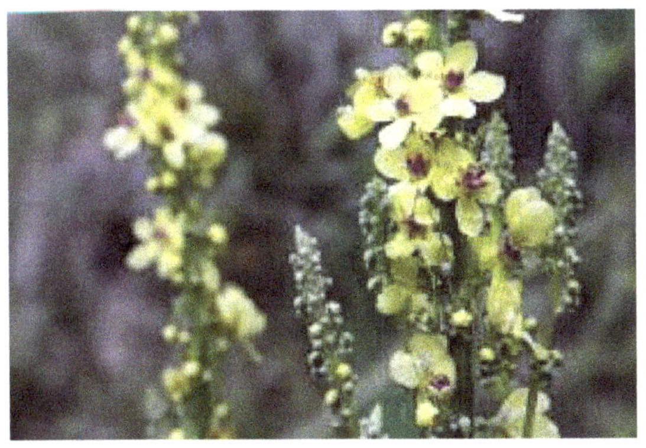

Watering Mullein Plants

This plant does not require an excessive amount of water. Once the plant begins to bloom, a minor increase in watering can be made. Otherwise, avoid keeping the soil consistently hydrated. You will inhibit growth.

- **Fertilizing Mullein Plants**

Mullein can be fed at your discretion; however, it is not required. Apply a slow-release, 10-10-10 fertilizer at the onset of the growing season if you are compelled to fertilize. This facilitates accelerated development and a profusion of blossoms.

- **Mullein Overwintering in the Garden**

Mullein is a biennial plant that is also resistant to freezing. This plant can withstand extremely low temperatures, as low as 5°C, which is considerably low for the majority of the United States and Europe.

Even though mulch can tolerate frost, it is still advisable to apply it prior to a frost. Reinforce the surrounding area of the plant with a stratum of fiber, branches, foliage, or bark. This provides insulation for the roots against freezing temperatures.

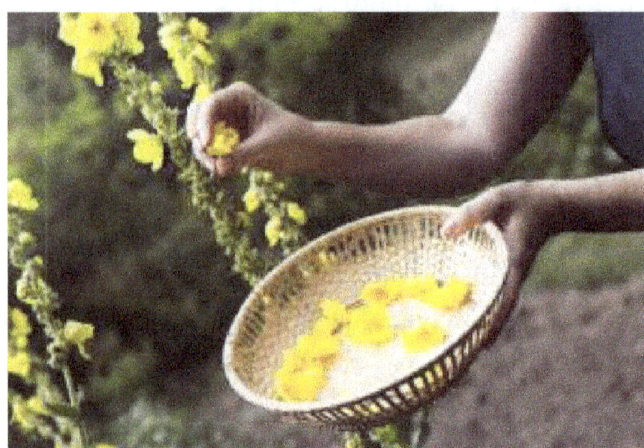

Harvesting Mullein

The collection of blossoms from mullein plants is possible from June to October. Doing so in the morning while the blossoms dry in the shade is optimalThe foliage gathered in the early hours of the day contains a greater concentration of essential oils. Ancestral harvests have a greater concentration of glycosides.

Herbalists assert that although mullein leaves are harvested during their initial year of growth, the efficacy of medicinal beverages can be enhanced by utilizing the leaves from the second year. The stalk and blossoms develop in the second year, and the blooms can be harvested daily as they open. In salads, the fresh foliage and blossoms make for a delectable addition. Additionally, the rhizome of the mullein herb can be harvested.

Once mullein has been harvested, it can be infused into medicinal herbal teas through the process of boiling water over either fresh or desiccated mullein leaves.

Utilize fresh, sizable mullein leaves to formulate poultices for the treatment of gout and joint discomfort. Mullein possesses a rich historical record of medicinal applications; therefore, seeking guidance from a certified herbalist is advisable when attempting to ascertain its proper utilization.

Dosing

The recommended dosage for mullein is as follows:

- **Tincture:** 2.5–5 mL of a 1:5 tincture (in 40% alcohol) three times daily.

- **Infusion:** To make an infusion, pour 1 cup boiling water over 2 teaspoons of dried mullein leaf or flower and infuse for 10–15 minutes. By passing through cheesecloth, every minuscule particle can be filtered out. Consume liquids three times daily.
- **Dried Herb:** 4–8 g of dried herb daily

How to Dry and Preserve Mullein

After spreading the flowers on a screen or paper towel, they can be left to cure naturally for multiple days. If they are to be used in the preparation of an infused oil or tincture, use them immediately. For several months, dried flowers for tea can be stored in brown paper sacks or jars out of direct sunlight. As soon as they begin to lose pigment, they also begin to lose potency.

Dried leaves present a greater challenge due to their substantial thickness. Pick the leaves only when they are entirely dry, with no moisture from dew or rain. It is beneficial to portion the leaves by cutting them in the center. Cut leaves into smaller pieces and air-dry on screens; alternatively, dehydrate them at 95 to 100 degrees Fahrenheit in a dehydrator. Additionally, cleansed, finely sliced roots can be dried in a dehydrator.

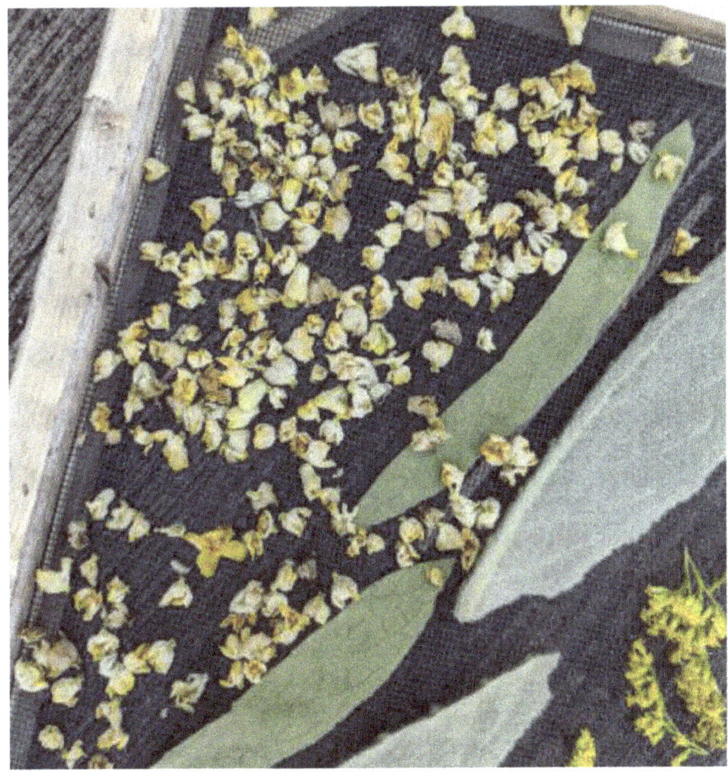

When not exposed to direct light, dried leaves can be preserved in paper sacks or jars for nine to twelve months, or until they begin to lose their color.

Salves and oil can be infused from both the foliage and the blossoms.

CHAPTER THREE

GINSENG

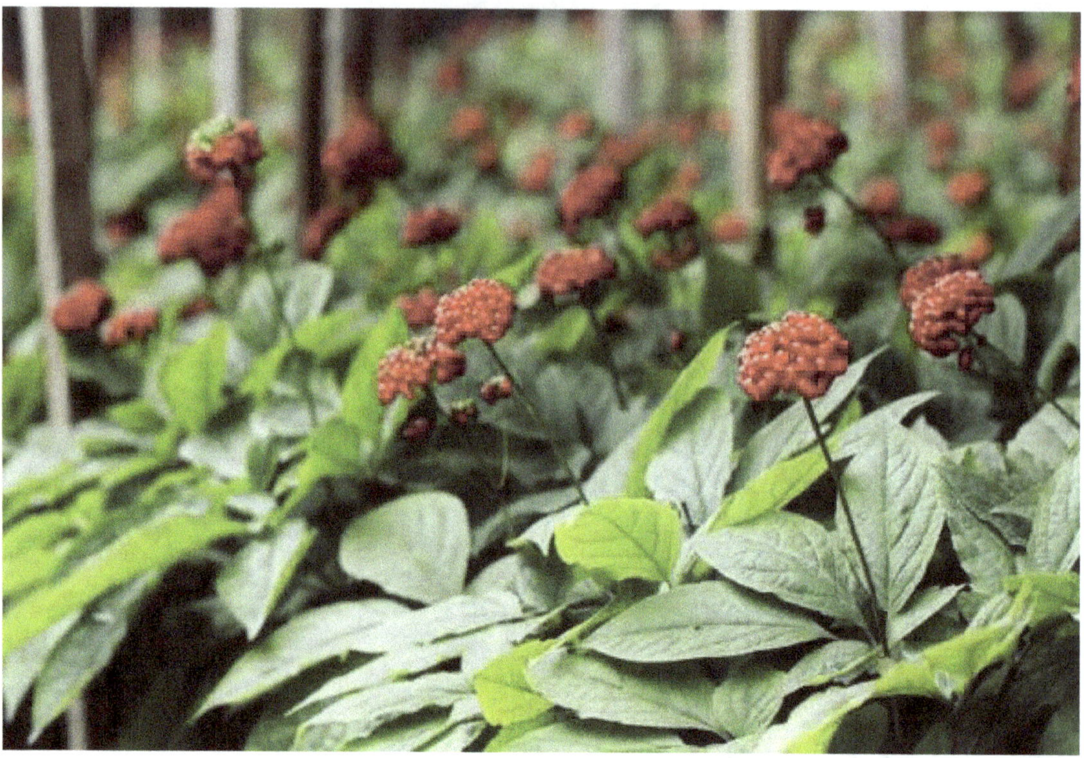

Ginseng is a perennial herbaceous root found in plants belonging to the Panax family, which includes ivy. Ginseng is extensively utilized in traditional medicine, particularly Native American and traditional Chinese medicine.

Red berries are the only byproduct of ginseng cultivation; the plant itself is grown for its roots. It is either cultivated or untamed ginseng, the former of which is found in its natural habitat in an organic state. Wild ginseng is endangered due to the excavation of its roots during the harvesting process; therefore, wild ginseng harvesting is strictly regulated in the United States and prohibited in some states. Although it is possible to cultivate and harvest ginseng at home, it is not required.

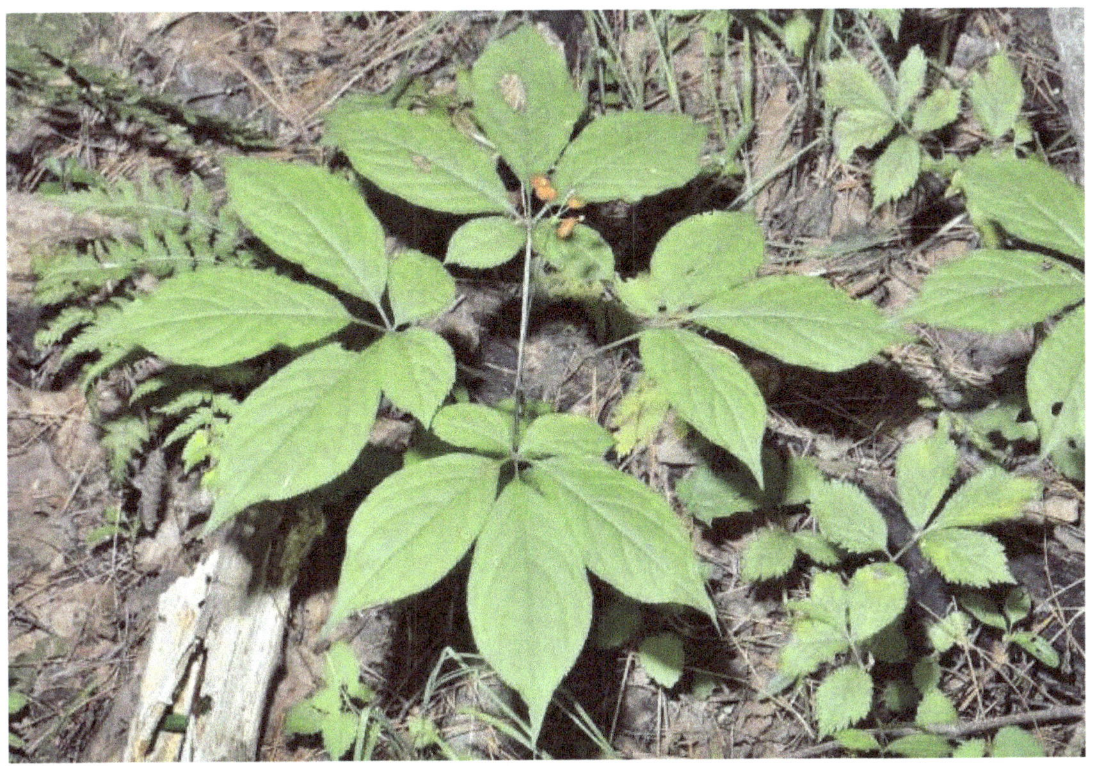

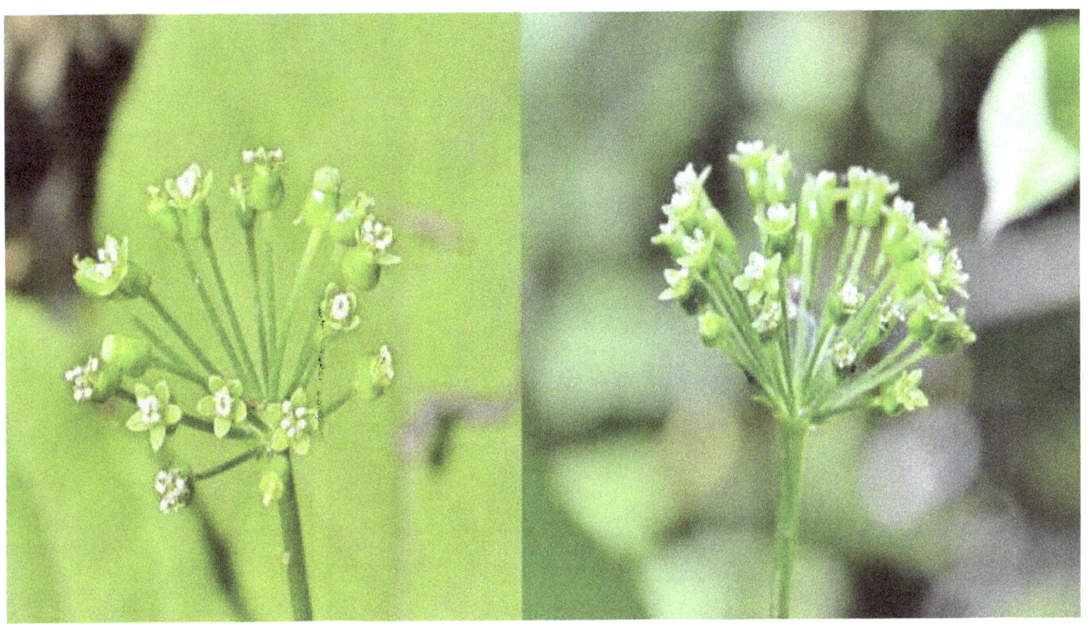

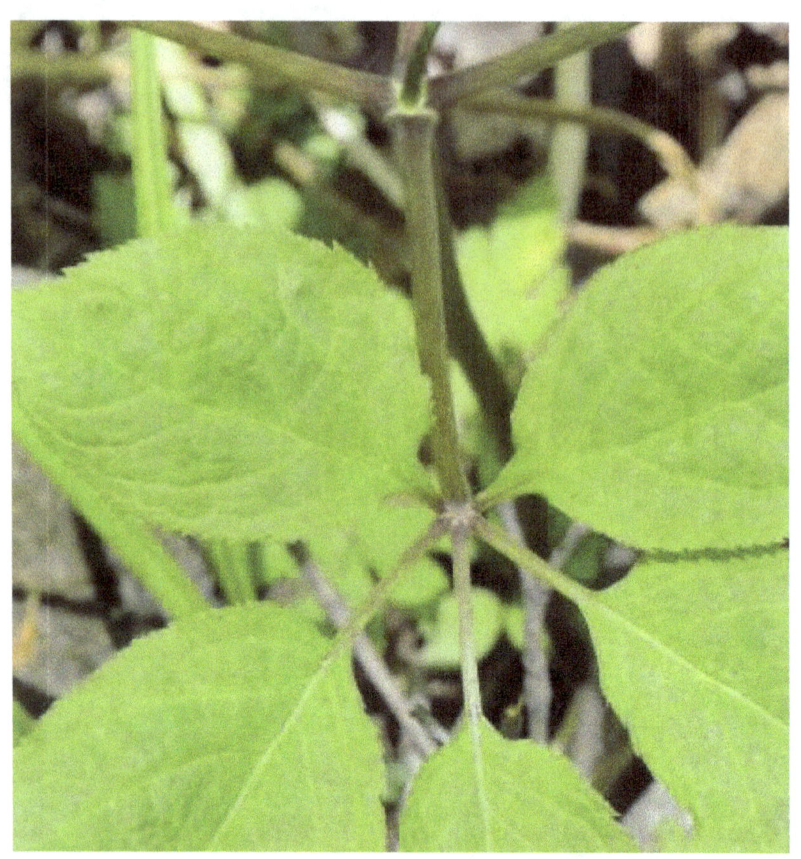

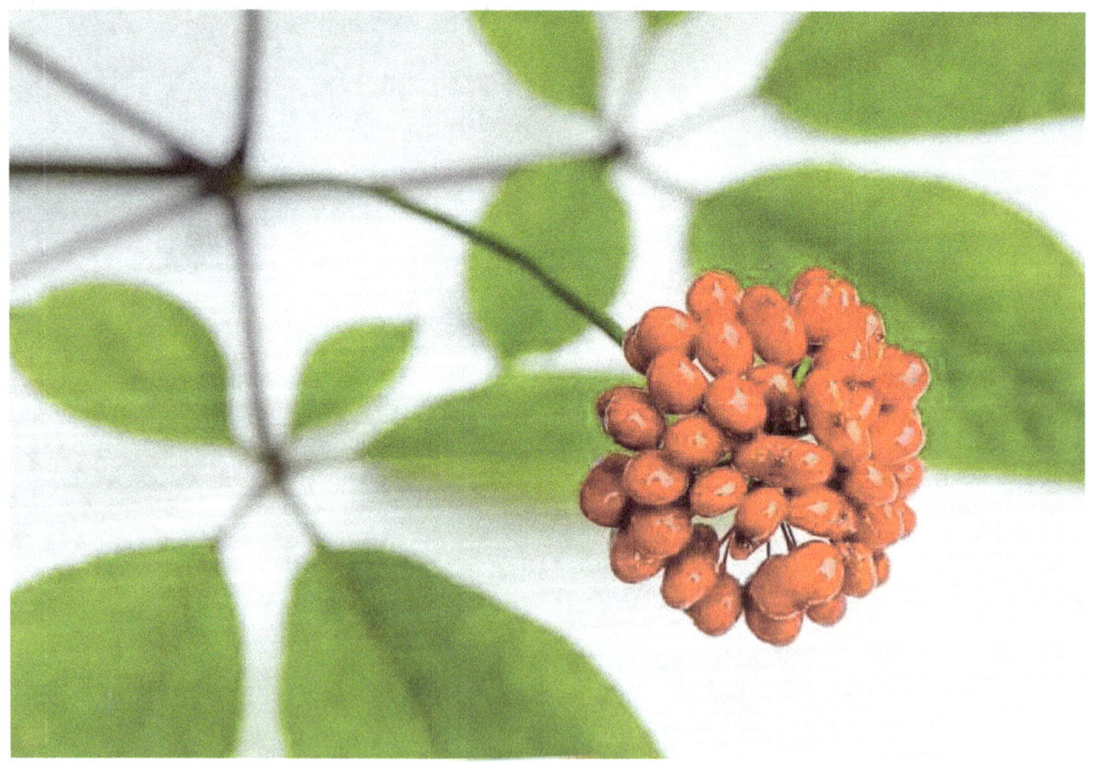

- **Leaves**

A number of palmately compound leaves atop the stem distinguish the roughly 25 cm-tall, fleshy-rooted perennial known as ginseng. The lower two leaflets are noticeably reduced in size in comparison to the three leaflets at the top, which possess an elongated oval shape.

- **Stem**

A number of palmately compound leaves atop the stem distinguish the roughly 25 cm-tall, fleshy-rooted perennial known as ginseng.

- **Fruits**

The fruit is a brilliant shade of crimson.

- **Flavor**

Ginseng possesses a light weight, a perpendicular-to-the-grain appearance, a thin consistency, and a delightful, viscous scent. It will have a slightly sweet flavor, followed by an astringent residue.

- **Root**

The mature root, which is utilized, has a length of 3 to 4 inches, a maximum thickness of 1 inch, and is commonly divided into two sections by circular crimping.

- **Edible part**

The desiccated root is frequently encountered in two forms: whole or sliced. Although ginseng leaf is not as highly regarded, it is still utilized on occasion. In Korean cuisine, ginseng is incorporated into an assortment of banchan (side dishes), guk (soups), tea, and alcoholic beverages.

Season

Red berries and at least three mature plants with five-pronged foliage should be collected. To ensure future ginseng plants, collect only during harvest season (September 1 through November 30) and sow seeds in close proximity to the harvested plant.

Habitat

Ginseng succeeds in dense hardwood forests characterized by nutrient-rich soils that are enriched locally.

The most common tree companions are sugar maple, white ash, and yellow birch; basswood is frequently encountered and can serve as a reliable indicator species.

Traditional Uses

Ginseng has been used for millennia in traditional Chinese medicine. With its antiviral, antioxidative, anti-inflammatory, anticancer, and antiobesity properties, this herb remains a well-liked medicinal component.

Research indicates that ginseng enhances circulation, fortifies the immune system, and provides protection against particular types of cancer. In addition, scientific studies have shown that the potent herb can improve diabetes treatments and reduce blood sugar levels.

Ginseng is a popular anti-aging herb utilized to support the mental health of older individuals on account of research demonstrating that it improves memory and learning.

Additionally, research has shown that ginseng exhibits analgesic and anti-inflammatory properties comparable to those of nonsteroidal anti-inflammatory medications (NSAIDs) and reduces inflammation in the body.

Ginseng Uses

As a dietary supplement, ginseng is offered in capsules, tea, dried botanicals, and powder form.

Ginseng is occasionally utilized as an additive in the production of commonplace products such as cigarettes, gum, toothpaste, soap, infant food, chocolates, and beverages. Both your individual inclinations and your financial requirements might influence the form that you select.

- **Root of ginseng**

Ginseng root is obtained from numerous plant species belonging to the Panax genus. The root is the botanical part that is commonly employed for medicinal purposes.

The root of ginger has a twisted, tan appearance. It is characterized by a stringed structure that extends to the lower extremities.

It is feasible to peel and consume the uncooked ginseng root. Furthermore, it can be consumed after being immersed in wine. Conversely, tea can be brewed by boiling the root.

- **Ginseng supplements**

A variety of forms of the ubiquitous dietary supplement, ginseng, are available

It's important to note that the FDA does not regulate herbal supplements, including ginseng. This may result in an incomplete understanding of the product's composition prior to consumption.

Gingesting ginseng supplements in the form of a tablet or capsule is permissible while drinking water. In general, these tablets consist of extract or pulverized root. They may consist of a diverse range of ginseng cultivars.

Ginseng root powder extract is soluble in an assortment of beverages. The concentrations of ginseng in the powder might exceed those present in the tablets or capsules.

- **Ginseng tea**

Ginseng is the substance from which ginseng tea is made. You may prepare your own beverages using powdered tea leaves or roots, or you may purchase prepared beverages.

- **Ginseng herbs**

Some research suggests that the health advantages of dried ginseng herbs may surpass those of fresh ginseng. While manual drying of ginseng is possible, the procedure can be quite challenging. Prepared dehydrated ginseng is commercially available at various retail outlets and online.

- **Ginseng Used in Food**

Ginseng is devoid of any inherent dietary origins. Ginseng is sporadically added to energy drinks and culinary products.

Additional applications of Ginseng consist of:

- Soups and stews
- Yogurt
- Oatmeal
- Stirred-fried foods
- Smoothies
- Beverages, juice, coffee, and tea are included.

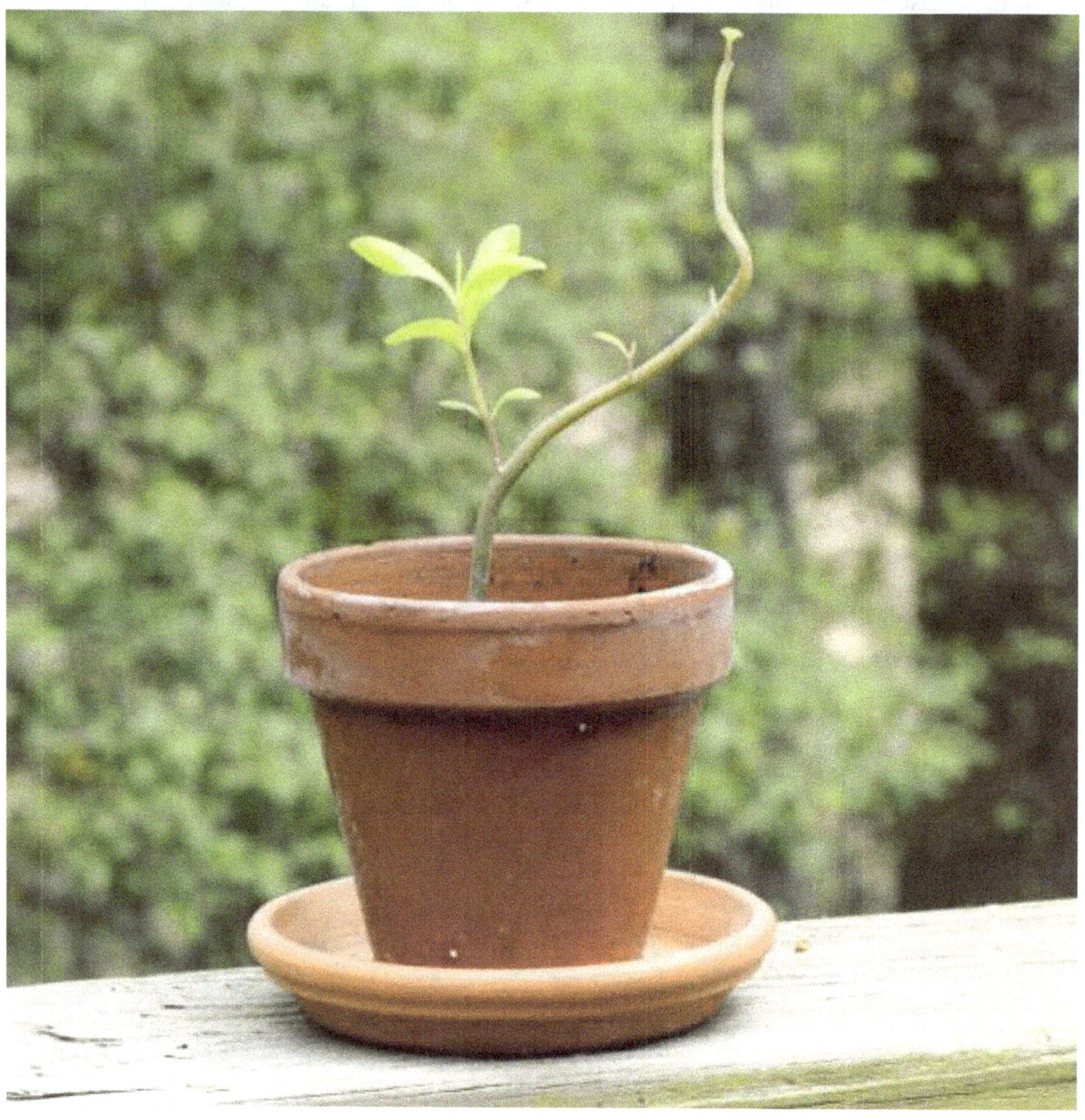

The most straightforward and secure method is to cultivate ginseng in a backyard that replicates its natural surroundings. Before starting ginseng cultivation at home, verify with state and local authorities that harvesting and cultivating ginseng is permissible in your area by conducting appropriate research.

Following verification that ginseng cultivation is permissible in your region, the subsequent guidelines will delineate the steps involved in carrying out this endeavor.

- **Select your own seeds.**

The simplest and most cost-effective approach for inexperienced ginseng cultivators to adopt is to procure stratified seeds from a nearby grower. This signifies the loss of the resilient outer layers of the seeds. While the price of these seeds is slightly higher than that of unstratified seeds, the rate of germination is considerably accelerated.

- **Select a location for planting and prepare it.**

Your growing area should have nutrient-rich, well-draining soil with a pH between 6.0 and 6.5. Please choose a location that receives minimal foot traffic and offers partial shade, or it can be shaded artificially if required. Remove any substantial pebbles or debris that could potentially hinder the development of your ginseng. Additionally, eight-inch plastic containers may be utilized to cultivate ginseng.

- **Plant your ginseng.**

By dispersing the ginseng seeds approximately one inch below the soil's surface and 14 to 20 inches apart, air circulation can be increased and the risk of disease reduced.

- **Do not rush.**

Up to 18 months may be necessary for the germination of ginseng seeds, and then another three to five years may pass before mature plants emerge. It is advisable to estimate the necessary time frame before considering the extraction of the subterranean components of the ginseng plant. Inspect the plant regularly for parasites and fungi as it develops.

How to Care

Gingeng plants necessitate minimal maintenance despite their extended periods of growth. The following is a summary of the necessary upkeep for your ginseng plant.

- **Give your ginseng water.**

Ginseng prefers a cool, damp environment. Water your soil frequently to maintain its moisture level; during periods of reduced precipitation, add additional water. Prevent root decay by ensuring that the plant is not excessively submerged in water.

- **Prune the planting site.**

In order to mitigate congestion, eliminate any branches or stems that encroach upon the area designated for planting ginseng from neighboring plants.

- **Keep it out of direct sunlight.**

It is optimal to store ginseng in areas that are partially or completely shaded. Ensure that the ginseng you are transplanting from a container outdoors is placed in a shady location.

- **Mulch**

When cultivating ginseng in a container or outdoors, supplement the soil with organic matter or leaf detritus to retain hydration.

- **Inspect for diseases and parasites.**

Animal damage or disease may be the cause of wilted foliage. Upon unearthing a wilted plant, scrutinize its roots for indications of gnawing or bite scars. Construct barriers or traps to prevent rodents and other vermin from causing harm to your ginseng site. Ginseng, which is also susceptible to leaf blight, may be managed by applying a thin layer of an organic fungicide.

- **Cautious of poaching**

Due to the protracted nature of ginseng cultivation, fully developed plants frequently become vulnerable to larceny or poaching. Certain cultivators opt to obscure their sowing sites by eliminating all aerial parts of their ginseng plant.

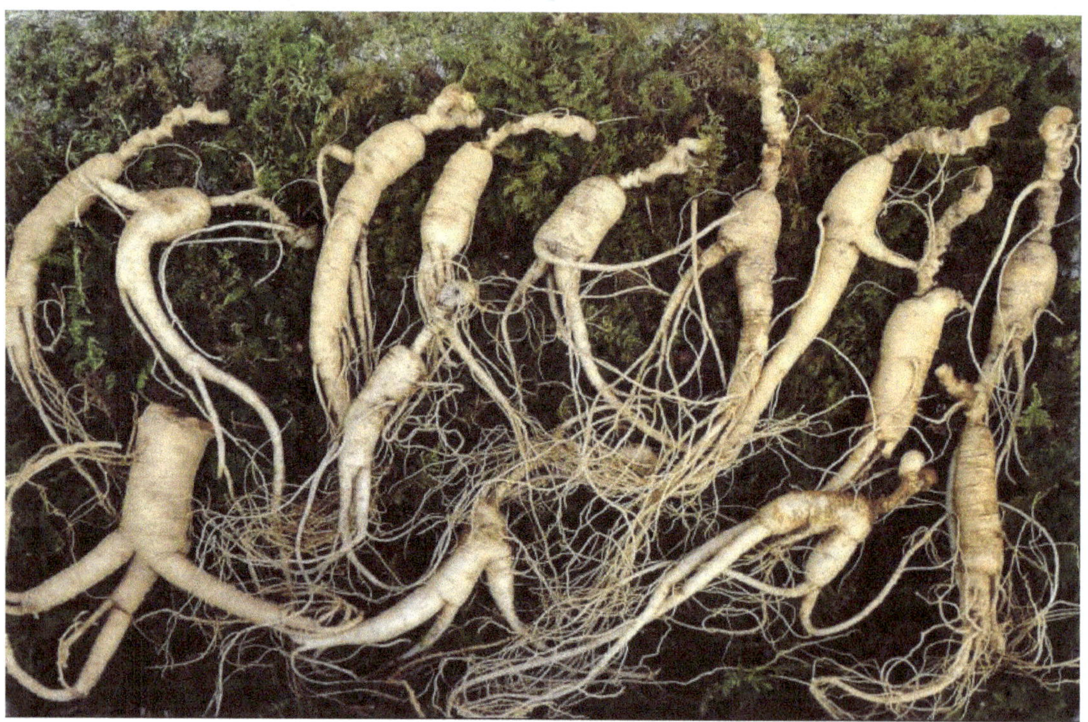

Harvesting Ginseng

The process of ginger harvesting necessitates meticulous attention to detail in order to prevent any damage to the roots.

- **Decompose the soil.**

Loosen the soil that envelops the ginseng plant and employ a gentle upward motion to extract any surplus soil from the plant's roots. To propagate additional ginseng, either harvest the mature fruit from the plant or replant it in the area where the root was extracted.

- **Rinse the ginseng.**

While taking precautions to avoid causing damage or rupture to the roots, gently rub the ginseng root with cold water to remove any excess soil.

- **Permit the ginseng to dry.**

Dry the ginger roots on a rack in a temperate location, away from direct sunlight, for a minimum of two weeks, or until the interior surface becomes translucent white.

Dosing

The type of ginseng, the quantity of ginsenosides in the supplement, and the intended use are some of the variables that affect Panax ginseng dosage.

There is no established dosage recommendation in place for Panax ginseng. Frequently, daily concentrations of 200 milligrams (mg) are utilized in investigations. Some sources recommend a daily intake of 500–2,000 mg of desiccated root-derived products. Dosages for capsules, when administered in divided portions, may range from 100 to 600 mg per day.

It is imperative to refer to the product label for guidance on administration, as dosages may vary. It is advisable to seek guidance from a healthcare professional before initiating Panax ginseng supplementation to ensure the usage is safe and effective.

Preserving Ginseng

Dried ginseng (root or powder) has a five-year shelf life when stored in an airtight container in a dry, dark location, such as a plastic bag or glass canister. Refrigerate newly harvested ginseng for a duration of two to three weeks.

CHAPTER FOUR

GINKGO BILOBA

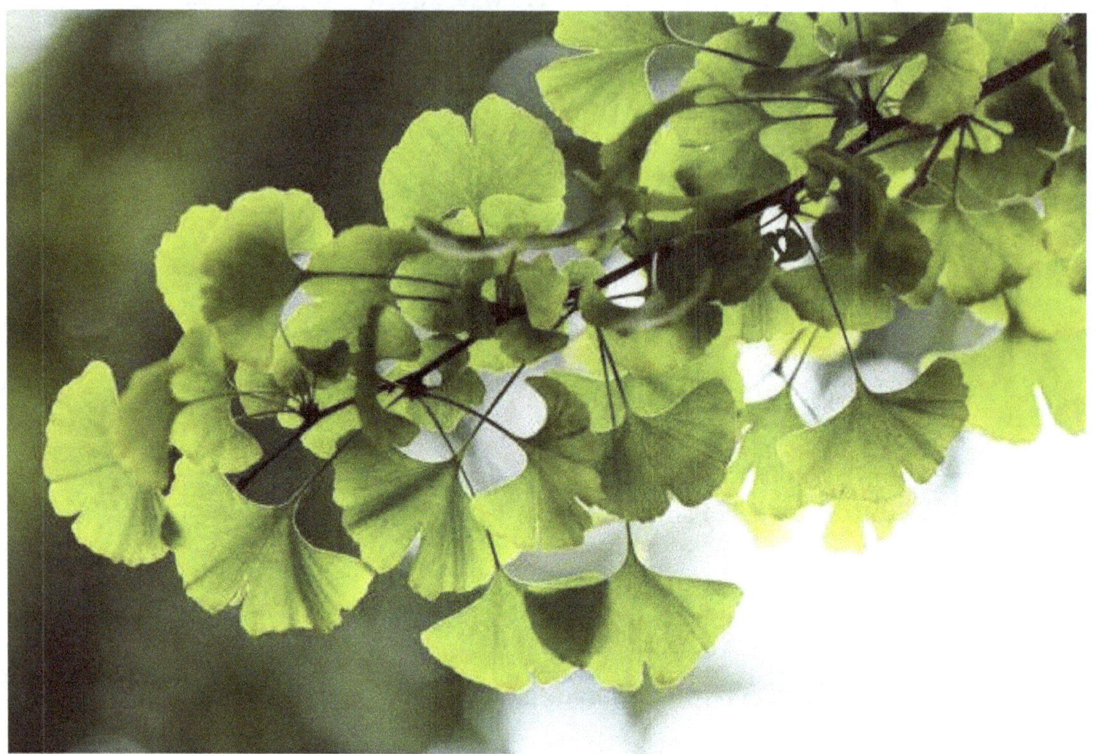

Ginkgo biloba, commonly known as ginkgo or gingko (/ˈɡɪŋkoʊ, ˈɡɪŋkɡoʊ/ GINK-oh, -goh), also known as the maidenhair tree, is a species of gymnosperm tree native to East Asia. It is the final extant member of the order Ginkgoales, which was established more than 290 million years ago.

Ginkgo fossils, which bear remarkable resemblance to extant species, were discovered during the Middle Jurassic period, approximately 170 million years ago.

Since the dawn of human civilization, the tree has been cultivated and continues to be planted extensively. Ginkgo leaf extract is commonly ingested as a dietary supplement; nevertheless, there is an absence of scientific evidence that disproves its purported ability to enhance human health or combat diseases.

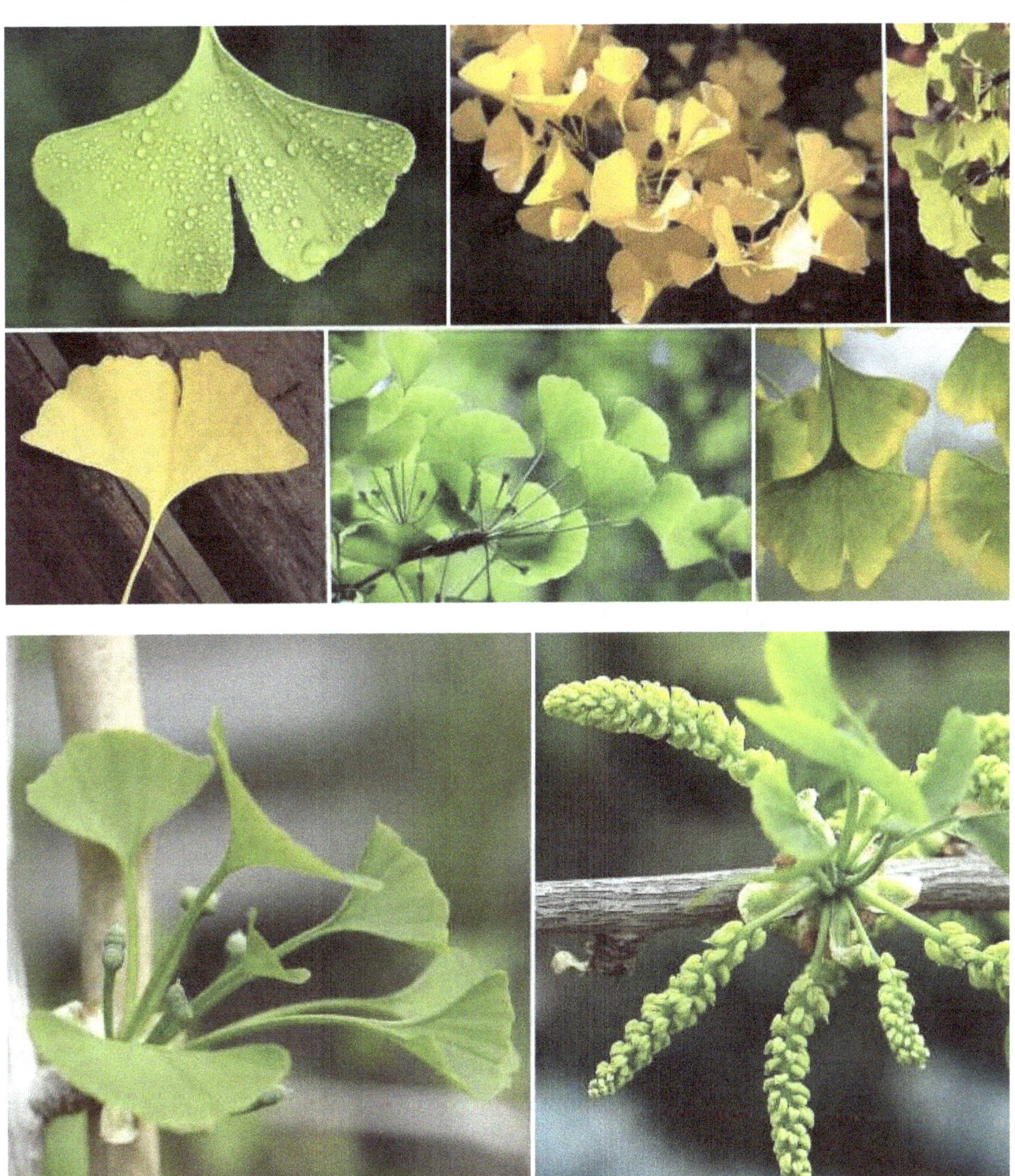

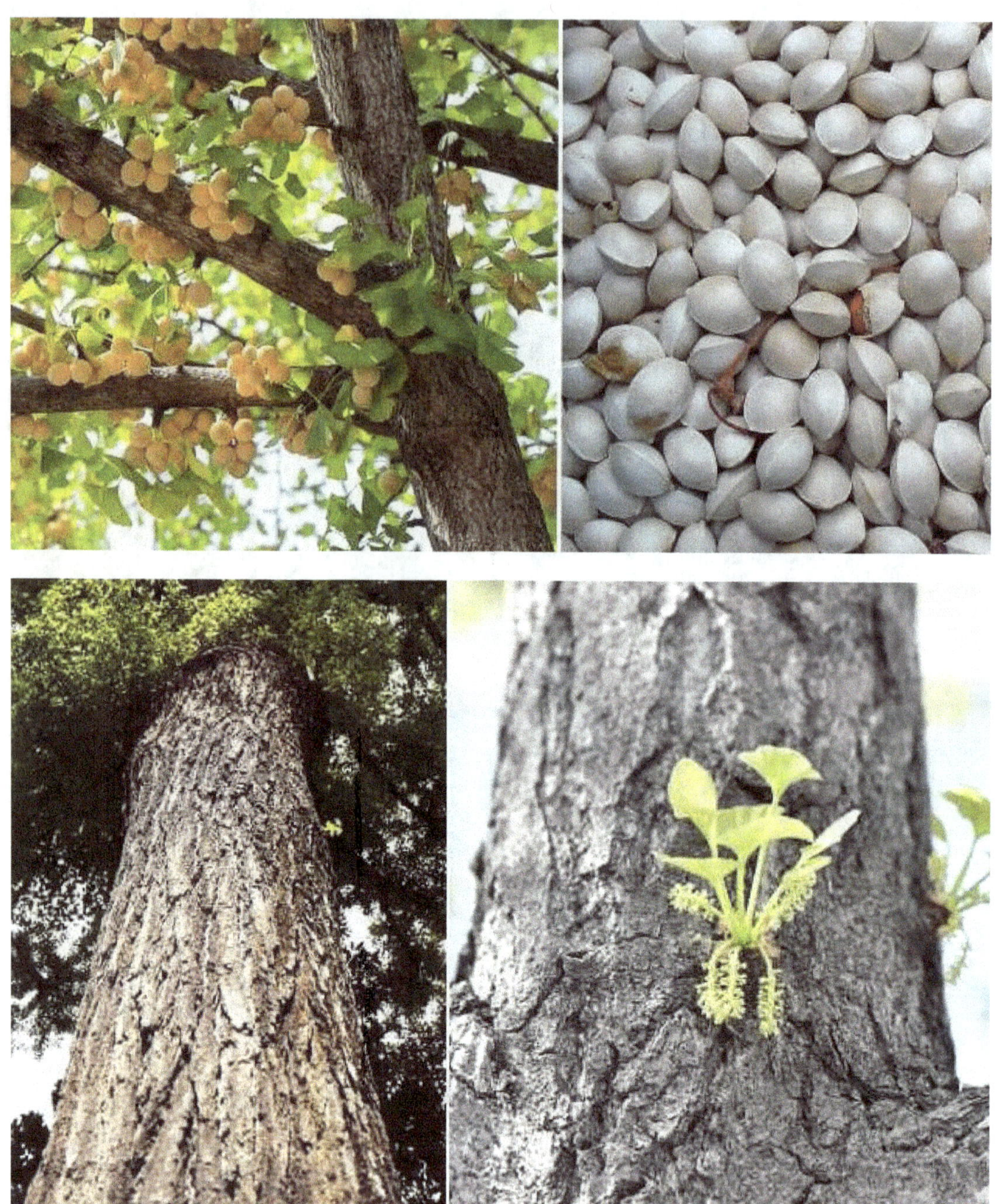

- **Trunk or bark**

Gingko fissured bark on mature trees is grayish in color, exhibits dense furrowing, and possesses a corky texture. The pallid wood was delicate and fragile. As a tree matures, its bark develops ridges and turns browner

- **Branches or twigs**

Ginkgo branch length is determined, similar to the majority of other tree species, by the development of shoots bearing leaves at regular intervals. "Spur shoots" (also known as short shoots) emerge from the axils of these leaves during the second year of growth.

Short branches are characterized by their unlobed leaves and exceedingly short internodes, which restrict their growth to a mere one to two centimeters over an extended period of time.

- **Height**

Gingko exhibits a minimum spread of 9 to 12 meters and a maximum height of 15 to 24 meters.

- **Needles and leaves**

Leaves of the ginkgo that are fan-shaped and bear on short, spur-like, yet significantly thickened stems resemble the leaflets of the maidenhair fern.

The leathery leaves can attain a maximal length of 8 cm (3") and can sometimes double in width to the same extent. Two parallel veins traverse each blade from the site of attachment of the long leafstalk and branch repeatedly in the direction of the leaf margins. A fissure in the center of the majority of leaves divides them into two lobes.

- **Flowers**

Flower production in gingko does not commence until the plants have reached reproductive age, which occurs between two and four decades of age. Specific trees engage in dioecious flowering, a reproductive process in which they exclusively produce male flowers and not female flowers. The flowering season for them occurs in April. Male flowers are catkin-shaped, yellow, and may attain a maximum length of 8 centimeters.

- **Flavor**

Herbal teas are comparable to Ginkgo biloba in that they contain the optimal combination of herbal flavor, astringency, woody nuances, and a greenish residue.

- **Fruits**

The kernel varies in length from one to two centimeters. The color of its fruit-like, succulent outer layer is a delicate yellow-brown.

While possessing an aesthetically pleasing appearance, this substance is made up of butyric acid (also known as butanoic acid) and, upon contact, emanates an odor reminiscent of rancid butter or regurgitation.

- **Edible parts**

While the seed itself is consumable in limited quantities, the fruit it encircles remains inedible. Throughout Asia, this widely used seed is employed in a variety of ways. The leaves are used to prepare a tea that is regarded as nourishing.

While leaves are generally safe to ingest in moderation, they do possess a significantly astringent characteristic.

The seed and leaf both contain an assortment of medicinal compounds. Numerous individuals extol the effectiveness of a leaf extract in facilitating the retention of memories.

Season

In spring, the leaves are a light green, but they turn a beautiful golden yellow in autumn.

Habitat

The tree demonstrates a predilection for sites that are exposed to direct sunlight. It exhibits the ability to flourish in loamy, gritty, and limestone substrates. Its occurrence is greater in areas distinguished by well-drained soil. It cannot undergo development when exposed to shade.

This tree, which has its origins in southeastern China, is presently cultivated in several countries, including regions of Canada.

Traditional Uses

For millennia, ginkgo leaves have been utilized for their medicinal properties. These include remedies for bronchitis, asthma, chronic fatigue, and tinnitus. While there is some conjecture regarding the potential brain-enhancing properties of ginkgo, further investigation is necessary to validate this idea.

The National Center for Complementary and Integrative Health states that the available evidence is inadequate to support the claim that ginkgo can effectively cure any ailment.

How to Use Ginkgo Nuts

After fifteen minutes at 350°F, encase the ginkgo seeds that have been pre-cleaned. In contrast to the resilience of black walnuts or pignuts, the shells of ginkgo nuts are easily fractured when subjected to a rubber mallet or tool.

Place the nut proteins between layers of dish towels to prevent the shells from bouncing around the room and crushing them. Subsequently, eliminate any paper envelopes that have become adhered to the nut meats.

By acquiring a green hue, cooked almonds enhance the flavor and aesthetic allure of soups, rice, and noodle dishes. To fully appreciate and discern the unique flavor and silky texture of ginkgo nuts, it is recommended to briefly fry them in oil and sprinkle them with salt.

For a refreshing beverage, these pair well with sake, wine, or lager. In addition, traditional Asian delicacies incorporate ginkgo seeds. Sweet cuisine is the process of integrating boiled, shelled almonds into desserts, cakes, and sweet stews.

Growing a Ginkgo Tree

Ginkgo trees exhibit remarkable resilience to severe wind, drought, and air pollution and flourish in Europe notwithstanding the absence of maladies. This robust tree is tolerant of both full sun and moderate shade conditions. Ginkgo trees exhibit a preference for moderately moist to arid soil, characterized by a pH value between 5 and 7. Soils that are nutrient-rich, deep, and permeable promote healthy development.

There are numerous cultivar configurations for gingko trees, including espalier, bonsai, umbrella-shaped, and spherical-high stems. The sowing spacing requirements of these plants differ depending on their growth pattern and upbringing. In all directions, specimen trees planted in a solitary position should be spaced 6–7 meters apart from other vegetation.

The planting distance for narrow varieties is two to three meters. The variety descriptions provided above detail the exact dimensions and growth patterns of each individual variety. Frost-sensitive young plants should be planted in March, just before their young foliage emerges.

- **Ginkgo planting in the garden**

In order to properly prepare the garden, it is necessary to loosen the soil and dig a trench of sufficient size to accommodate the ginkgo's deep roots. If deemed necessary, incorporate compost into the excavated soil as a supplementary nutrient source for the tree and a food source for microorganisms. Prior to introducing the root ball, verify that the planting aperture is balanced in depth with the initial pot.

Once the soil mixture has been inserted into the aperture, gently compact it around the root ball while forming a watering rim mound at the base. After driving two stakes into the ground in opposition to the wind and on opposite sides of the tree, affix the ginkgo to the tree using a rope. Thoroughly water the soil so that it can be redirected to the roots.

- **Establishing a potted ginkgo tree, or ginkgo bonsai**

Container cultivation over an extended period of time is only suitable for ginkgo varieties that mature slowly, such as 'Mariken'. Ginkgos can also be nurtured in the form of bonsai ornamentals. When shifting a ginkgo tree into a bonsai receptacle or container, employ a high-quality potting soil, such as our Plantura Organic All Purpose Compost.

It expeditiously provides essential nutrients to the plant subsequent to implantation and efficiently retains water to sustain the plant's hydration. To prevent waterlogging, line the bottom of the container with an approximately five-centimeter-tall drainage layer of expanded clay, gravel, or grit.

Place the tree on top of the potting soil, and compact the residual soil within the container. After the soil has been marginally compacted, apply substantial moisture to it. After two to three years have passed, transfer your gingko to a larger container.

How to Care

If the ginkgo has not yet developed substantial roots, it is necessary to provide it with water. It is crucial to consistently provide sufficient water to sustain plants in receptacles, especially in the midst of arid and scorching summer months.

However, exercise caution in order to avoid waterlogging. By incorporating a drainage layer of structural material before planting and choosing a container with a drainage opening, it is possible to facilitate the efficient drainage of excess water. Ginkgos are undemanding and low-maintenance garden inhabitants.

However, they require a tad more attention when grown in containers. Ginkgos grown in containers necessitate routine fertilization as a result of the limited accessibility of soil nutrients. Liquid fertilizers, such as our Plantura Liquid Houseplant Food, are optimal for this objective.

Commence applying the fertilizer on a regular basis in March. By adding it to the watering can, you will ensure that your ginkgo receives immediately and efficiently the two vital nutrients it needs to thrive—potassium and nitrogen.

Pruning is recommended for pruning-tolerant varieties of gingko trees in the spring. Crown training and thinning may be performed on a juvenile plant, if desired. Nevertheless, pruning is not mandatory.

On the contrary, the confined stature of bonsai ginkgo trees requires regular pruning. Immediately after developing, reduce a newly formed long branch with five to six leaves to two. When pruning bonsai, avoid creating large wounds whenever possible; thin, young branches should be pruned frequently.

Harvesting Biloba Ginkgo

Ginkgo berries are harvested using the same method as any other fruit: gently remove the berries from the branch using a harvesting pole or a gloved hand. As a result of the increased potential for skin contact with the fruit, attempting to scale a ginkgo tree may not be the most prudent endeavor.

Dosing and forms

Desiccated leaves, capsules, tablets, and liquid extracts are all viable options for incorporation into Ginkgo-infused beverages.

Studies have documented that adults consume 120 to 240 milligrams of the substance daily in divided amounts. It seems that a period of four to six weeks elapses before discernible enhancements become apparent.

Individuals who are the following should not consume gingko-biloba:

- Children
- Pregnant or nursing mothers
- Individuals with epilepsy
- Those who are on blood thinners

Patients with diabetes should not use gingko without first consulting a physician.

How to Store

The seeds of ginkgo must be refrigerated. They have an approximately one-week shelf life; dispose of them once an objectionable odor emanates.

CHAPTER FIVE

CHAMOMILE

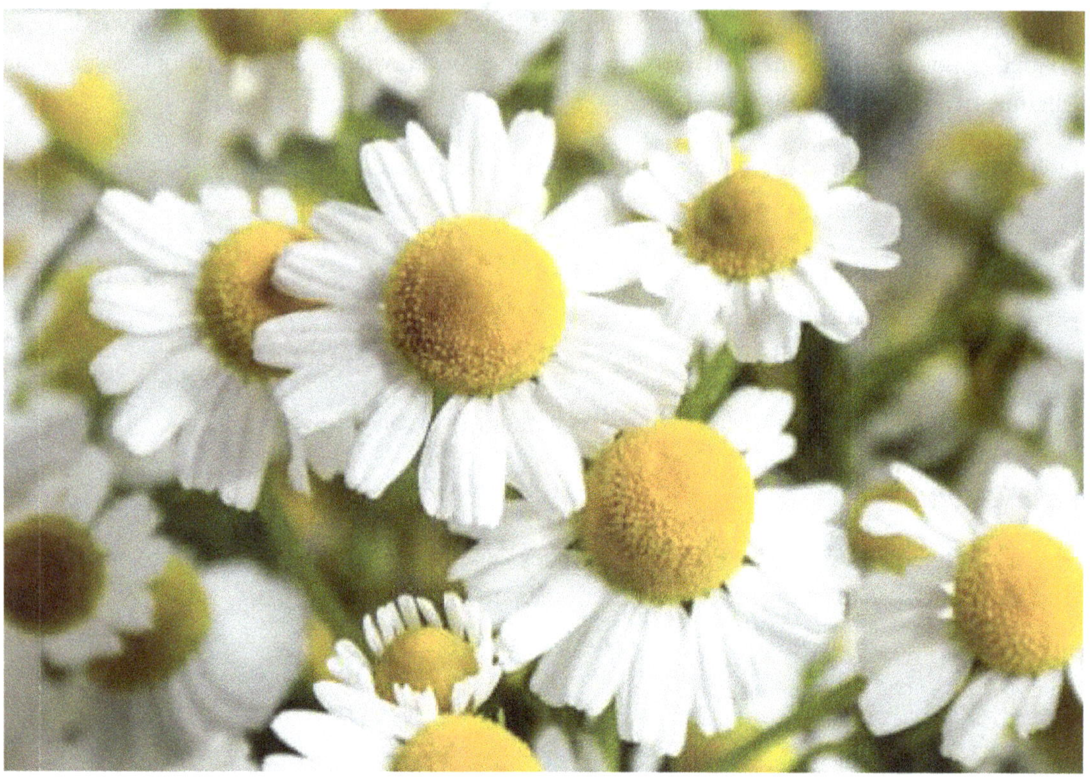

The spelling of the word "chamomile" differs between American English and British English. Several members of the Asteraceae family that resemble daisies are commonly known as KAM-myle or KAM-meel. Matricaria chamomilla and Chamaemelum nobile are two species that are commonly employed in the preparation of botanical infusions for beverages.

The potential therapeutic effects of chamomile supplements or consumables on medical conditions have received limited attention in research, despite its designation as the "king of herbs" in Hungarian.

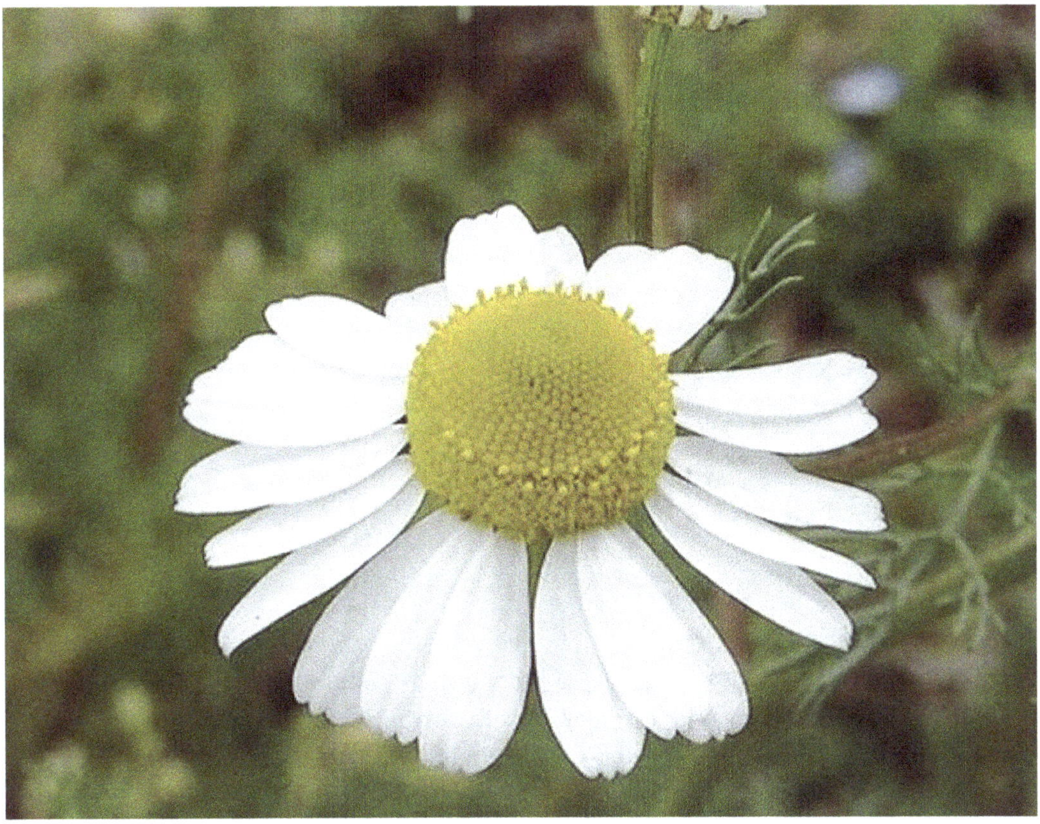

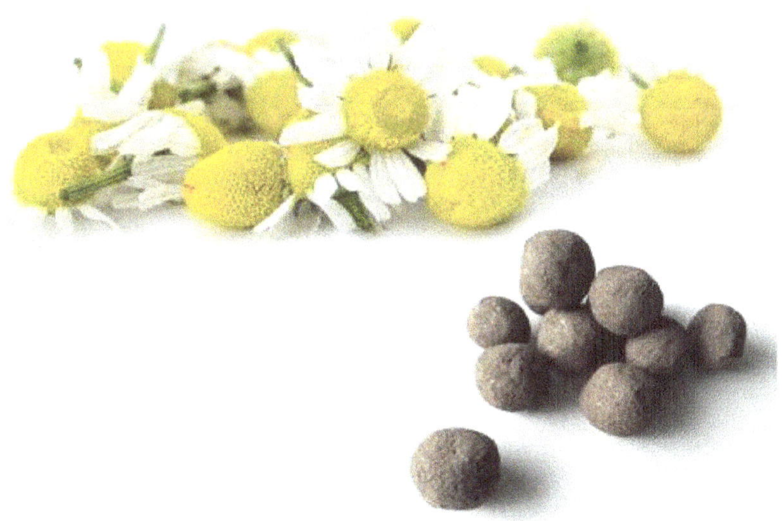

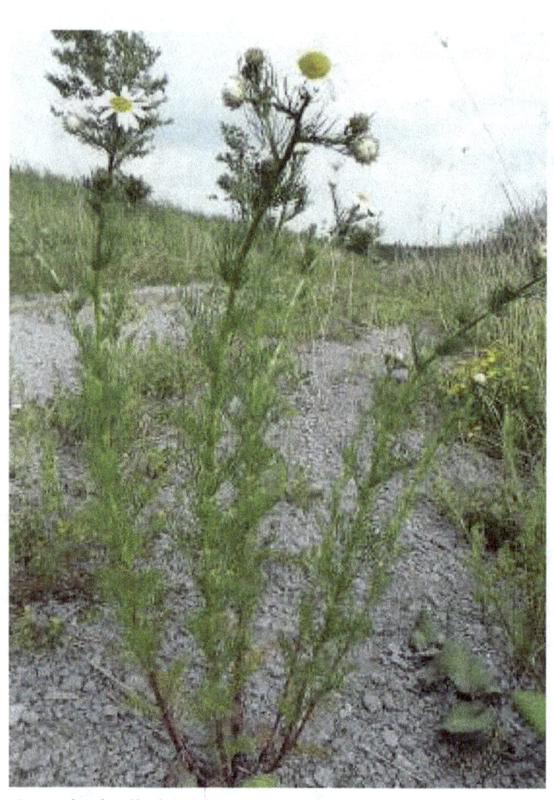

- **Leaves**

Feathered, green, and slender, reminiscent of fennel fronds

- **Flowers**

Daisy-like in size. Numerous white petals encircle a yellow center that is scaled.

- Stem

Sleek and smooth, measuring 15–60 cm in length

- **Fruits and seeds**

The flower stems of German chamomile dehydrate and become fragile; they also comprise minute brown elliptical seeds. Certain individuals obtain them with the intention of cultivating them indoors.

- **Aroma/Taste**

Chamomile, with its pleasant scent, imparts a unique aroma that is subtly reminiscent of pineapple. After a brief brewing process, the tea that emerges possesses subtle apple nuances and a sweetness reminiscent of honey.

- **Edible part**

The leaves, blossoms, and flowers of chamomile are all edible and appropriate for culinary preparation. However, utilization of the roots and stems is not customary. Additionally, animals can benefit from the medicinal properties of chamomile by consuming it.

Season

Spring and fall

Habitat

Disturbed areas, fields, and meadows

Traditional Uses

In the well-known herbal remedy of the rockies, chamomile is frequently employed to induce tranquility and alleviate anxiety.

The National Institutes of Health's National Center for Complementary and Integrative Health states that chamomile tea is "likely safe" to ingest. Additionally, it may be safe for brief periods of oral administration. The available information concerning the long-term safety of chamomile as a medicinal agent is inadequate.

Chamomile is utilized in Europe to reduce inflammation and edema, as well as to promote wound healing. Evident efficacy bolsters the herbal remedy's widespread appeal.

A 2016 study indicates that chamomile is an herb with numerous uses. It is commonly employed owing to its notable attributes, which include antioxidative, antimicrobial, antidepressant, anti-inflammatory, antidiabetic, and antidiarrheal.

Moreover, it facilitates the treatment of gastrointestinal disorders, premenstrual syndrome, knee osteoarthritis, and ulcerative colitis.

Ways to Use Chamomile

Are you ready to enhance your self-care routine by utilizing the extraordinary attributes of chamomile? Truly remarkable! In this analysis, we shall explore five straightforward yet influential approaches to incorporating this versatile herb into one's daily routine.

- **Chamomile Tea: A Soothing Herbal Infusion**

When confronted with the overpowering pressure and unpredictability of daily life, an individual might yearn for a moment of serenity and peace. There are instances in which an adequate quantity of chamomile tea is sufficient to elicit an internal state of serenity.

The Correct Procedure for Brewing Chamomile Tea

The process of concocting an optimal portion of chamomile tea is straightforward and soothing, inherently embodying a self-care routine. Follow the following steps in order to enjoy a delightful and serene herbal infusion:

- **Select chamomile of superior quality**

To commence, select chamomile tea that is of exceptional quality. Loose chamomile leaves and chamomile tea sachets are both available online and in local grocery stores. For optimal flavor and health benefits, choose organic, unadulterated chamomile blossoms that are free from synthetic fragrances and additives. I am in utter awe of these.

- **Water intended for boiling**

Bring fresh, frigid water to a simmer. The ideal preparation temperature for chamomile tea is approximately 200°F (93°C), which is slightly lower than its boiling point. When a kettle without a temperature control is not available, drizzle the chamomile with the chilled water once it has cooled for one to two minutes.

- **Determining the chamomile quantity**

In the case of chamomile flowers with sparse leaves, transfer 1 heaping teaspoon to an 8-ounce cup. Incorporate the chamomile into a teapot, infuser, or tea ball that possesses an integrated strainer. To utilize tea bags, merely pour one bag into the designated cup.

- **Infuse and pour**

Insert the chamomile tea bag or loose-leaf chamomile into the simmering water using an infuser. Tea should be steeped for five to seven minutes. The prominence of the sedative effects and the intensity of the flavor both increase in tandem with the steeping time. Nevertheless, an extended steeping period may result in the emergence of a pungent taste.

- **Remove tea bag or strain**

Pour the loose-leaf chamomile through a fine mesh strainer into a cup, or remove the tea bag or strain the chamomile after 5 to 7 minutes.

- **Add a touch of sweetness and garnish (optional)**

Chamomile tea can be garnished with honey, agave syrup, or sugar. In order to enhance the flavor, one might consider adding a lemon segment, a sprinkle of cinnamon, or a sprig of fresh mint.

- **Unwind and relish**

Ultimately, locate a comfortable location, take a seat, and relish the aromatic, soothing tastes of the ideal chamomile tea. Pause momentarily to completely appreciate the tranquility and warmth it imparts, and permit yourself to unwind and relax.

The advantages of chamomile tea

In particular, chamomile tea aids in the alleviation of stress and the attainment of interior tranquility. By enabling you to focus on what is truly essential—self-care—its calming attributes could potentially aid in the process of relaxation and the restoration of mental equilibrium. It is truly astonishing how something as simple as a steaming cup of tea can exert such an influence.

Among its numerous herbal advantages, chamomile tea possesses a notable capacity to enhance digestion. Have you ever encountered feelings of unease or dyspepsia following a substantial meal? Attempt to consume chamomile tea.

It has the potential to mitigate gastrointestinal distress and enhance overall gastrointestinal health. Moreover, its absence of caffeine renders it a caffeine-free beverage that can be consumed at any time of day without concern for disrupting sleep.

When you next encounter feelings of being overwhelmed or digestive issues, keep in mind that a cup of chamomile tea has the potential to be a profound remedy. This calming herbal infusion serves as an optimal remedy for various circumstances, be it the desire to alleviate abdominal distress or to find solace amidst a tumultuous environment.

This way of incorporating chamomile into one's self-care and self-love routine is among the simplest, illustrating that sometimes the simplest solutions are the most effective.

- **Chamomile Bath: A Luxurious Home Spa Experience**

As a result, one might perceive existence as superfluous, necessitating a momentary respite. It is possible that an individual is contending with the intricacies of everyday life or has endured a prolonged phase of stress.

Regardless of the situation, a chamomile bath is an invitation to pause and rediscover one's inner tranquility. Additionally, a few simple elements and some "me time" are adequate; neither a luxury spa nor expensive treatments are necessary.

Upon entering the water, the calming properties of chamomile will begin to promote relaxation of the muscles. A tranquil ambiance is fostered through the harmonized fusion of the soothing aroma and the moderate temperature, which encourages repose and relaxation.

Methods for Creating the Ideal Chamomile Bath

Do you feel equipped to DIY a chamomile bath? The following items will be necessary for you:

- Four to six packs of chamomile tea bags or one cup of loose chamomile blossoms
- A balmy, water-filled bathtub
- To enhance the therapeutic and calming effects, one may contemplate the incorporation of lavender essential oil, Epsom salt, or a few drops of chamomile essential oil as discretionary supplementary components.

To prepare the chamomile bath, steep the tea leaves or loose chamomile blossoms in a large kettle of boiling water for approximately ten minutes. After straining the chamomile-infused water (if using dispersed flowers), transfer the solution to a tepid bath. None of the optional ingredients should be added at this time. Soak in the tub while in a state of comfort, permitting the therapeutic properties of the aromatic and soothing waters to take effect.

Remember that at this juncture, you should engage in self-compassion and relaxation. Create an atmosphere of tranquility within your chamomile bath through the execution of a sacred ritual, which may include activities such as meditating, lighting candles, or listening to soft music. Create an atmosphere of heightened awareness by focusing on the pleasurable sensations of comfort, relaxation, and the invigorating fragrance of chamomile that surround you.

Consequently, why not indulge your bathtub and benefit from the therapeutic properties of a chamomile bath? Participating in self-care and demonstrating well-deserved self-love is a straightforward and efficacious approach. In the end, you have earned it!

- **Enhancements to Self-Massage and Meditation with Chamomile Essential Oil**

Have you ever contemplated how self-massage could be improved to be more nourishing and utilized as a straightforward, organic approach to enhance one's meditation routine? The solution is readily apparent in front of you. By augmenting your meditation and self-massage practices, the calming aroma of chamomile essential oil can perform marvels.

As an effective meditation aid, chamomile essential essence is utilized. The serene fragrance of this substance aids in establishing an atmosphere of tranquility and serenity, promoting cognitive relaxation, and nurturing a sense of self-connection.

By embracing the calming fragrance of chamomile, individuals can facilitate the surrender of distracting thoughts and shift their focus to the present moment. By facilitating a more robust mind-body connection, chamomile essential oil encourages the cultivation of deep self-awareness and self-love and enhances performance during meditation sessions.

Self-massage is an additional self-care practice that can be substantially enhanced through the application of chamomile essential oil. Body massage oil, which is infused with chamomile, promotes emotional equilibrium and relaxation via a comforting, nurturing sensation in addition to nourishing the skin. People can fully participate in the therapeutic action of manipulating their own hands thanks to the calming atmosphere that the delicate chamomile scent creates. Your act of massaging your body while nourishing your spirit is a beautiful demonstration of self-love.

The Optimal Method for Employing Chamomile Essential Oil in Self-Massage and Meditation

Including chamomile essential oil in one's massage and meditation regimens is a straightforward process. The subsequent guidance will aid you in commencing the process:

- To facilitate meditation, a few droplets of chamomile essential oil can be easily combined with an aromatherapy inhaler or diffuser. As you prepare your meditation space, inhale the soothing fragrance, allowing it to guide you into a state of profound inner serenity and relaxation.
- To perform a self-massage, blend a few droplets of chamomile essential oil with your preferred carrier oil, such as sweet almond oil or jojoba (which is my personal favorite!). While applying the mixture to your epidermis, be sure to concentrate on areas that are tense or require additional attention. It is imperative to establish a mindful connection with one's body and show it the reverence and kindness that it merits.

Hence, it is advisable to integrate chamomile essential oil into one's self-care routine. It is a straightforward yet effective way to enhance one's meditation and self-massage practices due to its tranquil aroma and numerous beneficial properties. It is precisely by nurturing one's psyche as well as one's body that one can achieve self-love and self-care.

- **Uncover Your Natural Beauty with Chamomile Skincare**

The world of hygiene can undoubtedly induce a sense of being overwhelmed. A multitude of products assert themselves as conducting miracles, thereby posing a challenge in discerning which ones to truly believe.

If you are tired of deciphering lengthy ingredient lists and prefer a more natural approach to sanitation, chamomile may be the answer you've been seeking. Through promoting self-care and fostering an admiration for one's inherent beauty, this unassuming blossom bestows substantial advantages on the hair and complexion.

One might question the mechanism by which chamomile could manifest such a significant impact on the hair and epidermis. It is rich in anti-inflammatory and antioxidant compounds, making it a natural and gentle method of skin care and nourishment.

Additionally, chamomile is versatile, as it can be incorporated into numerous formulations to address an extensive range of skin and hair concerns. It can alleviate psoriasis and eczema, as well as reduce the erythema and irritation that accompany inflamed or irritated skin.

Moreover, chamomile's anti-inflammatory properties can be extraordinarily beneficial for the scalp, alleviating dryness, dandruff, and irritation. Moreover, its tranquil and calming aroma can augment the sense of relaxation and indulgence experienced throughout one's hair and skin care regimen.

Are you inclined to integrate chamomile into your regimen of natural cosmetics? The subsequent recommendations outline potential incorporations of chamomile into skincare and hair care routines:

- **Chamomile Face Steam**

Combine a handful of dried chamomile flowers or a few droplets of chamomile essential oil in a large bowl filled with hot water. Lean over the basin while draping a towel over your head in order to capture steam. As you profoundly inhale, allow the chamomile-infused steam to purify your skin and enlarge your pores.

- **Chamomile Face Mask**

Combine honey and plain yogurt with a few drops of chamomile essential oil or chamomile tea to create a soothing face mask. Allow the mélange to sit on your face for fifteen to twenty minutes following application, prior to rinsing. You will notice that your epidermis is renewed and revitalized.

- **Chamomile Hair Rinse**

Permit a kettle of potent chamomile tea to cool before applying. After shampooing, apply the chilled tea to your hair as a final rinse. An overtly gradual process of lightening one's hair can achieve the appearance of sun-kissed skin, diminish dandruff, and provide relief to the scalp.

- **Chamomile-Infused Products**

Maintain a watchful eye out for personal hygiene products that contain chamomile as a vital constituent. These may comprise cleansers, toners, and moisturizers, offering chamomile-infused ready-to-use formulations for increased efficacy and convenience.

By incorporating chamomile into your hair and hygiene routines, you are not only nurturing your skin and hair but also engaging in self-love and self-care. Presently is the moment to commemorate the radiant and lovely being that you are by embracing chamomile's natural attractiveness.

- **Chamomile for Sleep: A Route to Peace and Serenity**

While lying in bed, the events of the day consume your thoughts, rendering slumber an unattainable ideal. You are twisting and turning in bed once more. A positive development is that chamomile, our preferred blossom, has the potential to function as the sleep aid you have been looking for: it induces a sense of calm and relaxation before bed and improves the overall quality of your sleep.

Chamomile has been employed for centuries as a natural sleep aid, and for good reason. The calming properties of this substance facilitate relaxation and the release of anxieties that might be hindering sleep during the night by soothing the body and mind.

At the same time, chamomile may provide alleviation to those who suffer from migraines or headaches. The substance's intrinsic analgesic properties may alleviate tension migraines and promote a more tranquil sleep.

The Optimal Sleep Benefits of Chamomile

Interested in integrating chamomile into your evening routine? The subsequent recommendations outline potential uses of chamomile to promote a more tranquil sleep:

Before retiring for the evening, prepare a cup of chamomile tea for consumption. When combined with the soothing properties of chamomile, the thermal energy of the tea will contribute to physical relaxation and mental serenity, ultimately facilitating the descent into slumber. Furthermore, incorporating tea into one's bedtime routine can function as a comforting bedtime custom that alerts the body to the impending arrival of sleep.

- Produce a chamomile sleep mist by combining water and a few drops of chamomile essential oil in a spray bottle. Prior to bed, mist the mist onto your pillow and bed linens. By illuminating your boudoir with the calming scent of chamomile, you will be able to drift off to sleep effortlessly.
- Consider utilizing a chamomile-infused eye pillow: Place a few droplets of chamomile essential oil or flaxseed and dried chamomile flowers inside a small fabric pouch that has been stuffed over the eyes while you retire to bed. Chamomile's calming aroma and mild pressure will aid in the alleviation of stress and the promotion of relaxation.

Encourage the use of chamomile in bedtime meditation. Spend a few moments engaging in meditative meditation while sipping chamomile tea or inhaling the fragrance of chamomile sleep mist. By directing one's attention towards the breath and permitting any worries or concerns to dissipate, one creates an environment conducive to a tranquil and rejuvenating slumber.

Not only is integrating chamomile into your bedtime regimen a simple way to demonstrate self-compassion and care for yourself, but it is also an all-natural and efficacious approach to enhancing the quality of your sleep.

Therefore, the next time you experience difficulty falling asleep, keep in mind that chamomile can assist you in attaining a state of tranquility and peace. Sweet slumber!

- **The Use of Chamomile in Food**

Chamomile is generally harmless for use in foods, according to the FDA. In teas, dried blossoms of German chamomile are frequently utilized. More frequently, Roman chamomile is employed as a delicate flavoring in various beverages and dishes.

Chamomile may be incorporated into salad dressings, baked products, jams, and candies. It is also employed as a decorative garnish and to flavor ice cream and cocktails.

- **Incorporate chamomile into your daily life to be more self-careful and loving.**

To conclude, chamomile is an authentic resource for self-love and self-care. This multipurpose blossom has the potential to alleviate tension, enhance digestion, promote relaxation, and bolster emotional health. In addition, it functions as a bedtime support and a natural cosmetic supplement for the skin and hair, aiding in the process of falling asleep peacefully.

It is widely recognized that the pursuit of self-care does not adhere to universal principles, and what proves effective for one individual may not resonate with another. But isn't it incredible to consider how a substance as uncomplicated as chamomile could have such an impact on our existence? By integrating chamomile into our daily wellness regimens and embracing its manifold advantages, we can foster an enhanced sense of self-compassion while healing our physical, mental, and spiritual beings.

Now is the moment to apply what you have recently acquired! Whether you choose to prepare a calming cup of chamomile tea, indulge in a tub infused with chamomile, or devise your own chamomile self-care routines, keep in mind that you are deserving of every bit of affection and attention that is given to you.

Therefore, why not experiment with chamomile and experience the calming embrace of this captivating blossom? Best wishes as you progress in developing a deeper sense of self-compassion and affection.

Have fun with it!

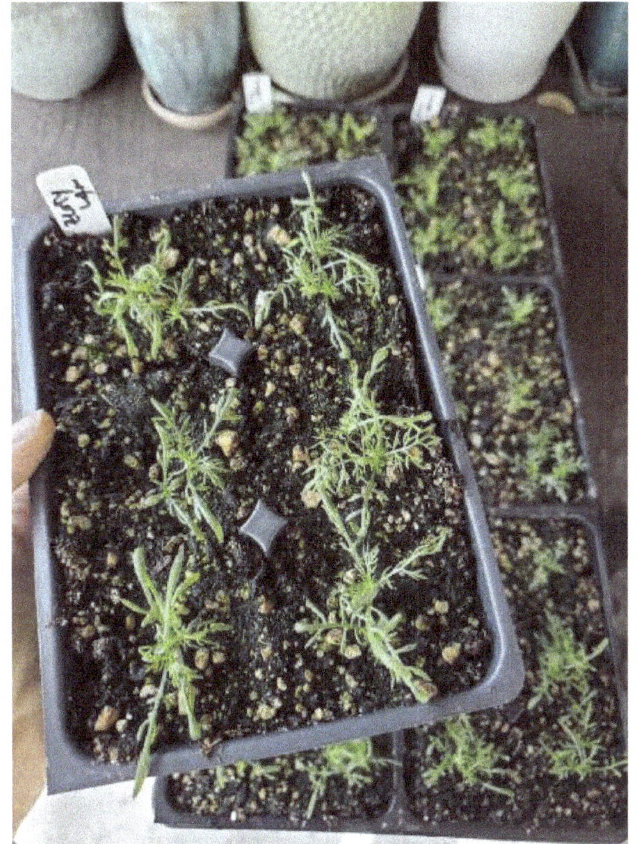

Chamomile, a delightful asset to any garden, is well-known for its pleasant aroma and numerous health benefits. Chamomile cultivation is a relatively straightforward and advantageous endeavor. Regardless of one's level of expertise as a cultivator, the subsequent recommendations will aid in facilitating the robust growth of chamomile plants.

Selecting the Ideal Position

In terms of environmental suitability, chamomile flourishes in both direct sunlight and moderate shade. A site that obtains a minimum of six to eight hours of sunlight on a daily basis is considered ideal.

- **Irrigation**

Verify that the soil at the designated location possesses sufficient drainage. Due to the fact that chamomile abhors "wet feet," persistently saturated soil can result in root damage.

Moisture and soil

- **Soil Type**

Chamomile exhibits optimal growth in alluvial soil with a neutral pH. Despite this, this adaptable herb can thrive in a wide range of soil conditions, provided it has sufficient drainage.

- **Watering**

Although chamomile plants develop resistance to drought once they become established, consistent watering is crucial during their initial phases of growth. It is of the utmost importance to avoid overwatering; permit the soil to dry slightly prior to adding additional water.

Planting from seeds

- **When**

Sow chamomile seeds directly into the soil or indoors six to eight weeks prior to the last anticipated chill, in late spring.

- **Spacing**

Seeds may be lightly broadcast onto the soil when sowing. Once the seedlings have fully developed and emerged, reduce them to a distance of 10–12 inches.

- **Depth**

In order for chamomile seeds to germinate, they require light by being gently compacted into the soil without being completely covered.

Maintenance and care

- While chamomile is generally resistant to pests, aphids and mealybugs should be consistently monitored. You can employ a natural insecticidal soap or a vigorous stream of water to ward them off.
- Organic mulch applied around the circumference of chamomile plants can aid in moisture retention and pest control.
- When the plants are young, consider cutting back the crowns to promote bushier development.

How to Care

Minimal maintenance is required for chamomile plants. After being cultivated, they acquire a moderate drought tolerance. It is essential to maintain consistent watering for plants grown in containers while also ensuring proper drainage to prevent the entrapment of roots in waterlogged compost.

In order to maintain bushy growth and prevent chamomile plants from becoming lanky, regular pruning is required.

How to Harvest a Chamomile Flower

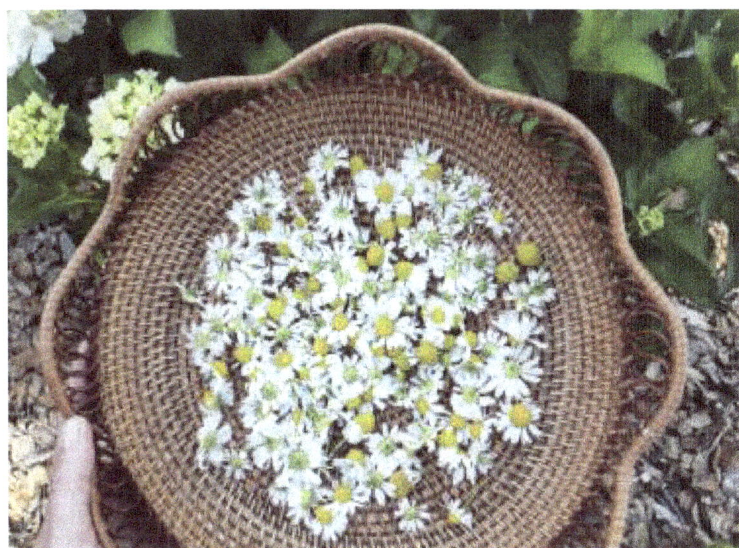

The process of harvesting chamomile is uncomplicated: simply use your fingertips to remove the daisy-like flowers from the upper portions of the stems. They dissipate instantly with a pleasant explosion. The implementation of a specialized selecting cultivator streamlines the chamomile harvesting procedure, especially when a significant quantity is being cultivated.

It is not inappropriate to harvest chamomile. Additional blossoms will develop as more are harvested. Chamomile demonstrates uninterrupted flowering from spring to autumn and in regions characterized by moderate, frost-free climates, even in the dead of winter. As of February, we continue to harvest chamomile from plants that were planted last autumn, despite a minor deceleration in production.

To maximize the potency of essential oils and the flavor of tea, harvest chamomile flowers while they are still in their youthful stages.

This occurs shortly after the flowers have fully opened, but before the centers undergo inordinate enlargement and the petals begin to droop inward. The majority of herbalists advise harvesting chamomile in the early morning before the sun and daytime heat degrade the delicate essential oils.

Dosing

A universally accepted dosage for chamomile is not feasible, owing to the extensive range of formulations available.

Prior to utilizing chamomile, individuals who are pregnant or nursing, have a preexisting medical condition, or are currently taking medications should consult their physician. It could potentially impede the efficacy of the supplements or medications you are consuming.

It is advisable to seek the advice of a pediatrician before introducing any type of chamomile supplement to children or neonates.

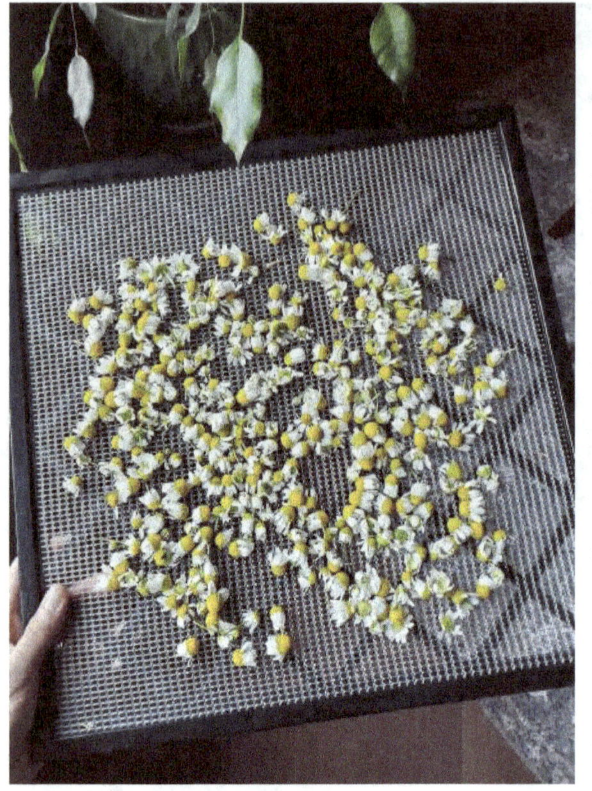

By allowing chamomile flowers to dry naturally or in a food dehydrator, they can be dehydrated. To prevent the addition of unnecessary moisture, which would prolong the drying process and increase the probability of mildew growth, chamomile is not rinsed subsequent to harvest.

Arrange the chamomile flowers in a single layer on a screen, in an airy container, or on an herb drying stand in a warm, dry, arid location. If required, augment the flow of air by incorporating a fan. Flower mold growth may occur prior to complete drying if the air is excessively humid or if the blossoms are not distributed sufficiently.

A food dehydrator is an ideal apparatus for dehydrating chamomile, especially in preparation for oil infusions, tinctures, or salves or for long-term storage.

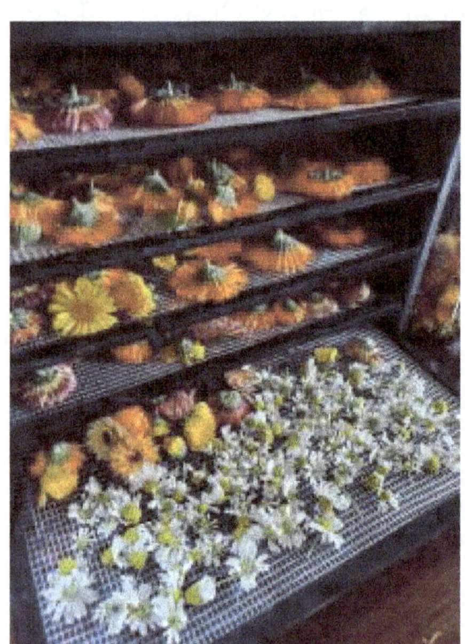

When producing oils or salves, it is critical to utilize flowers that are completely dried, as any residual moisture in the flowers can accelerate the growth of mildew or the deterioration of the final product. For chamomile to retain its medicinal and beneficial compounds, it must be dried at an exceedingly low temperature.

We maintain our dehydrator at a minimum temperature of 110°F (or the lowest setting accessible) for a minimum of 24 hours. Although the drying process can be accelerated at higher temperatures, it is not recommended to dry chamomile flowers in an oven.

After the chamomile has dried completely, place it in an impermeable container (e.g., a glass container with a lid) and store it in a cool, dry, dark location. The advantageous attributes, aroma, and flavor of the substance will endure for a period of one year at that particular site.

CHAPTER SIX

YARROW

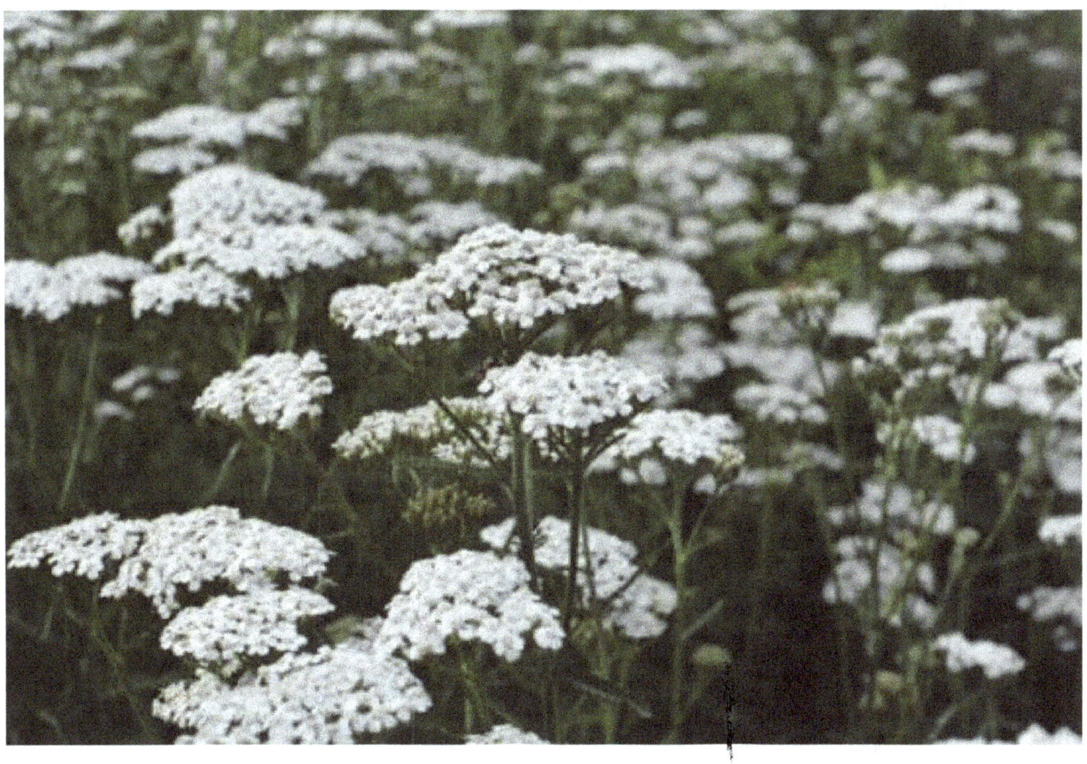

An herbaceous perennial, yarrow (Achillea millefolium), is characterized by its elevated stems, fern-like foliage, and clusters of minuscule flower heads that develop into circular blossoms. Yarrow plants exhibit an extended flowering period spanning from early spring to late autumn, with an average height of one to three feet. Yielding resistance to pests and adversity, yarrow is a resilient plant that is indigenous to Asia, Europe, and North America.

The flower heads adorn a garden, flower container, or lawn with vivid yellow, red, white, or pink blossoms. Devil's nettle, milfoil, old man's pepper, thousand-seal, and thousand-leaf are all common names for yarrow. Yarrow cultivars such as 'Paprika,' 'Cerise Queen,' and 'Moonshine' are well-liked.

Yarrow, being a pollinator-attracting wildflower, elicits the attention of birds, butterflies, and bees. Yarrow is commonly regarded as a companion plant due to its ability to restore essential nutrients to the soil, including calcium, potassium, and phosphorus. Yarrow blossoms are simple to maintain as cut flowers due to their tall stems; they also make for exquisite centerpieces.

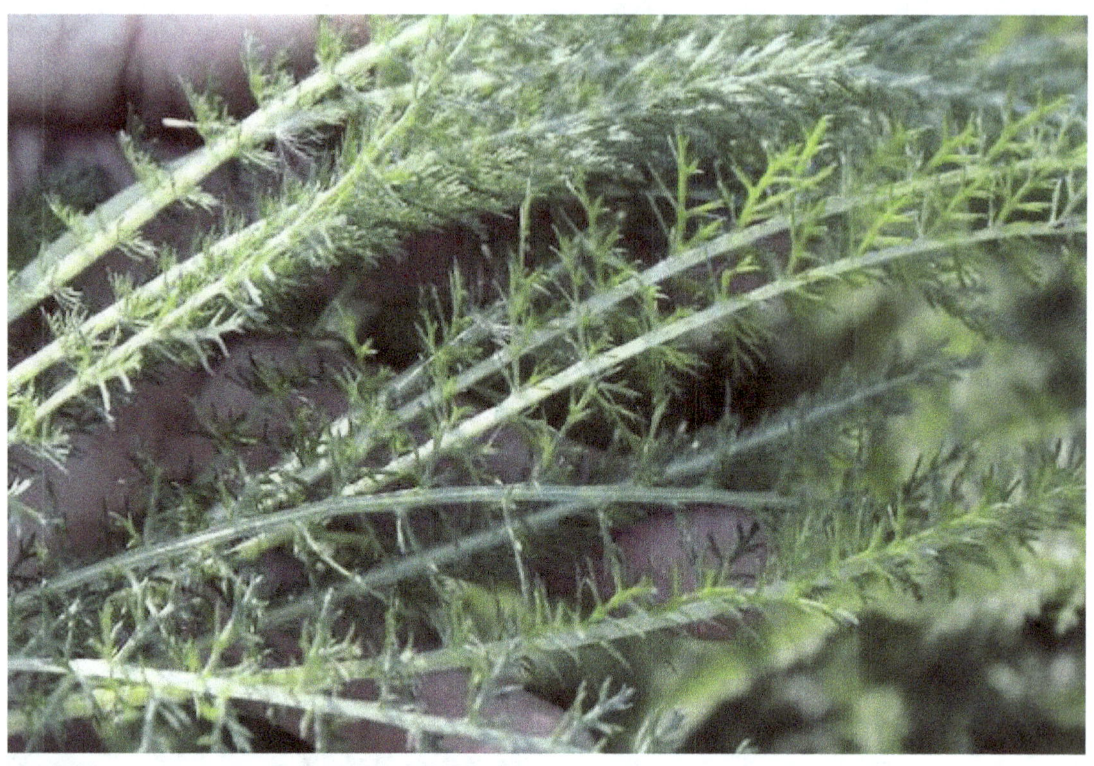

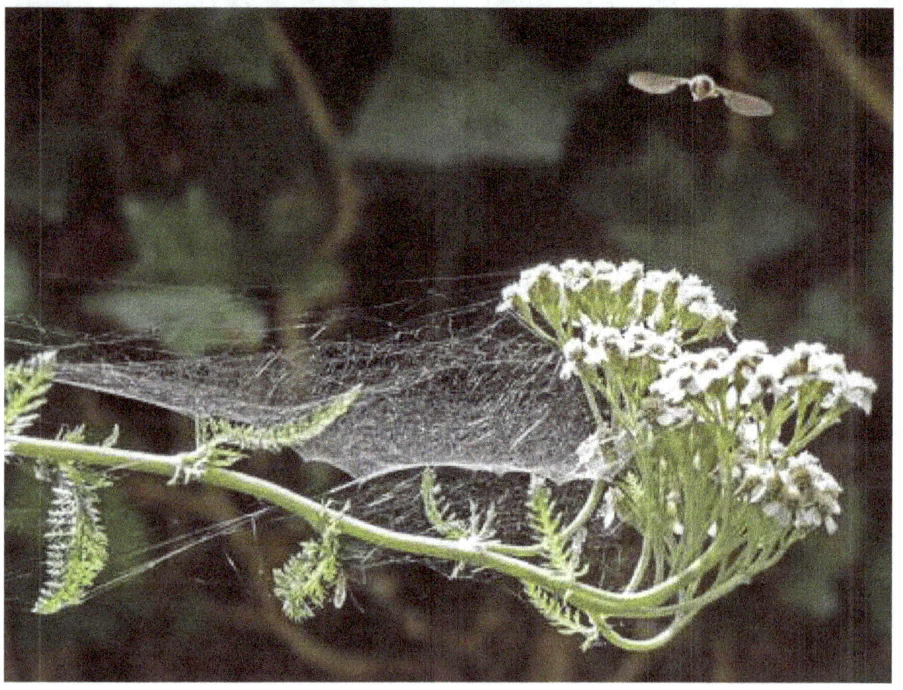

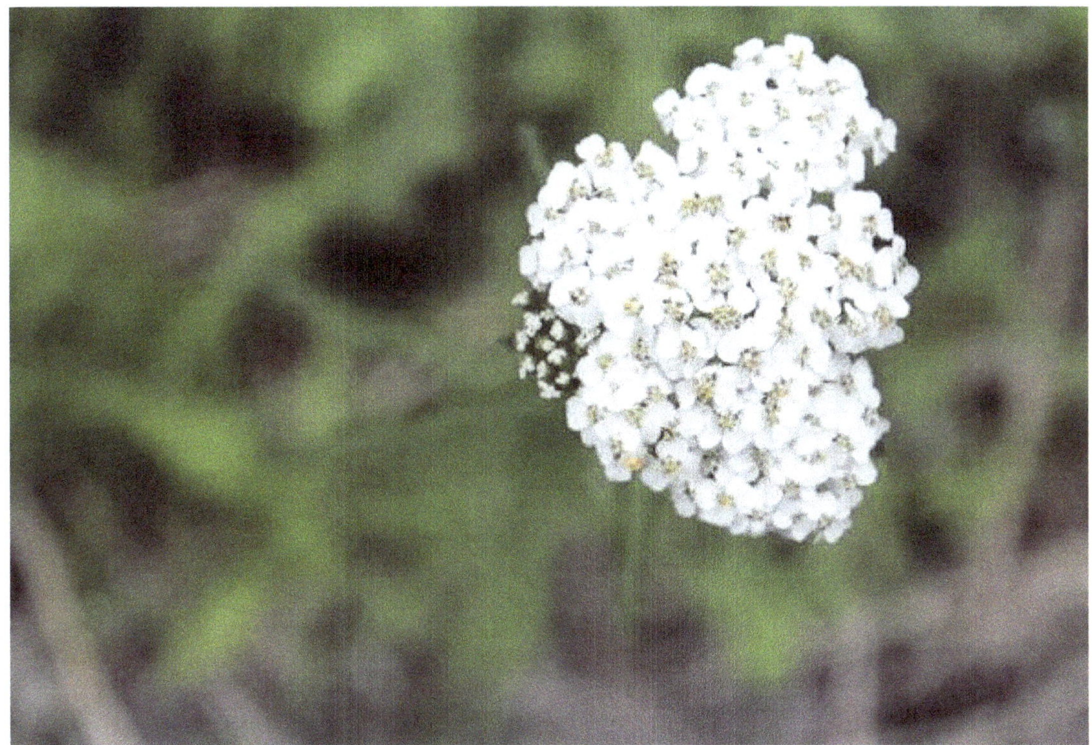

- **Leaves**

Green leaves that are either bipinnate or tripinnate encircle the tiny stem in a feather-like fashion.

- **Flowers**

From June to September, a cluster of tiny white to pink flowers is arranged in an umbrella-like formation.

- **Taste**

It is virtually tasteless, with a hint of medicinal undertones.

- **Smell**

An aroma is produced when the leaves or blossoms of yarrow are subjected to crushing. Others may interpret it as a blend of camphor and chamomile, whereas some describe it as a delicately aromatic fragrance.

- **Fruits**

The cypsela are the diminutive fruits resembling achenes.

Season

Depending on the region, yarrow blooms from late spring to early autumn on average. Flower colonies proliferate during this period, attracting pollinators including bees and butterflies.

Habitat

Gardens, roadsides, fields, meadows, and virtually any other area where grass thrives

Medicinal Uses

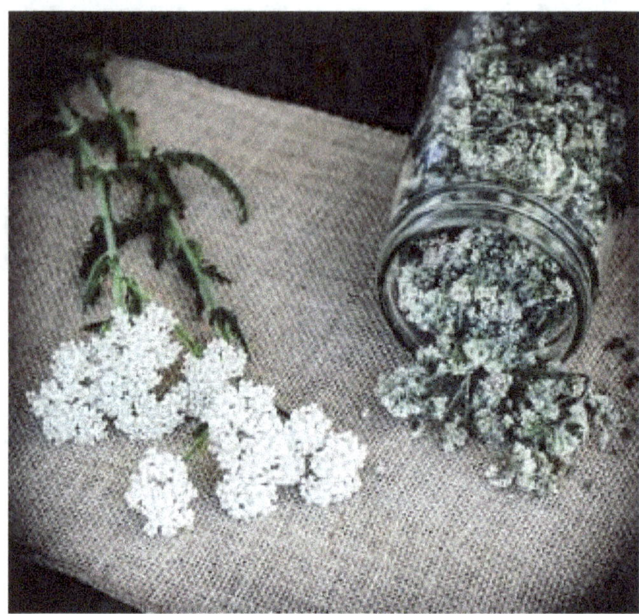

Regarding foraging for medicinal plants, yarrow is among the most significant to be conscious of.

Yarrow is a valuable herb to possess due to its antiseptic, astringent, antimicrobial, and anti-inflammatory attributes, which render it applicable to a diverse array of maladies.

To halt bleeding, yarrow leaves may be utilized as a poultice or ground into a styptic powder. Applying the styptic powder, derived from yarrow leaves that have been dried and pulverized, directly to the site of bleeding is recommended.

Due to its remarkable coagulating properties, yarrow has been employed historically to staunch hemorrhaging on the battlefield throughout periods of conflict.

Yarrow supports the reproductive system and enhances circulation by regulating menstruation and balancing the monthly cycles of women. Additionally, it supports digestive health.

An herbal salve formulated from yarrow can also be utilized to promote the healing of minor scrapes and wounds. Additionally, yarrow is renowned for its capacity to assist in temperature regulation in cases of fever.

Both consuming a cup of yarrow tea and immersing in a yarrow leaf soak will provide relief. This is an excellent method for reducing a toddler's or infant's body temperature.

As a relatively potent diuretic, yarrow tea can be consumed for medicinal purposes to treat infections of the urinary tract. Because yarrow tea is so bitter, a homemade tincture that is highly concentrated may be a more appetizing way to consume the herb.

What is Yarrow used for?

Yarrow is used in a considerable variety of cultural and traditional contexts. Some frequent applications of yarrow include:

- **Medicinal Purposes**

Yarrow has been utilized in traditional herbal medicine for a very long time. There are multiple medicinal properties attributed to it, such as anti-inflammatory, antispasmodic, and analgesic effects. It has been utilized to promote wound healing, alleviate menstrual discomfort, and treat digestive issues and illness.

- **Herbal infusions and teas**

The flowers and foliage of yarrow may be utilized in herbal infusions or brewed into herbal teas. It is commonly believed that the aromatic characteristics of these beverages impart calming and soothing qualities.

- **Culinary Uses**

Yarrow may be incorporated into specific dishes as a culinary herb. The aromatic, slightly astringent leaves and flowers can be used to enhance the flavor of salads, soups, stews, and herbal vinegar infusions.

- **Insect Repellent**

Yarrow is renowned for its insect repellent properties, which include the ability to deter mosquitoes and flies. Certain individuals employ yarrow-infused sprays or perfumes as an all-natural insect repellent.

- **Dyeing**

Yarrow has been used as an organic dye source. Yellow, gold, or greenish dyes may be produced from its flowers when utilized in the dying procedure.

Other applications consist of:

Thus, we proceed to the preparation and consumption of yarrow. Listed below are several yarrow recipes that call for common yarrow:

- **Herbal Yarrow Tea**

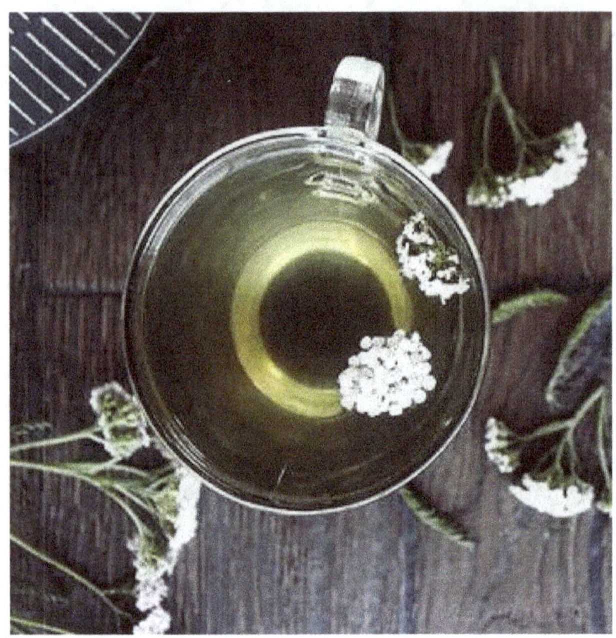

Ingredients

- Combine 1 cup of hot water with 1 tablespoon of dried yarrow flowers and foliage.

Instruction

- In a cup, combine the desiccated yarrow flowers and leaves. Allow them to steep in heated water for five to ten minutes. If desired, strain the tea and consume it unsweetened or sweetened with honey. If you have them, embellish with fresh yarrow flowers and fronds.

- **Yarrow Salad**

Ingredients

- Tomatoes, cucumber, red onion, feta cheese, mixed salad greens, fresh yarrow leaves and flowers, salt, pepper, and lemon juice.

Instruction

- Additionally, the yarrow flowers and foliage, salad greens, cherry tomatoes, cucumber, and red onion should be washed and dried. Incorporate each of the components into a salad basin. To prepare the dressing, combine olive oil, lemon juice, salt, and pepper in a separate bowl using a whisk. Olive oil should be drizzled over the salad, then tossed gently. Serve with crumbled feta cheese on top.

- **Vinegar Infused with Yarrow**

Ingredients

- Yarrow flowers and fresh foliage, along with white wine vinegar.

Instruction

- Thoroughly cleanse and dry the yarrow flowers and foliage. Cover the contents of a clean glass container with white wine vinegar. Shake the jar intermittently while storing it in a cool, dark location for two to four weeks with the lid securely sealed.

- Strain the vinegar following the infusion period in order to eliminate the yarrow plant material. Infuse vinegar infused with yarrow for use in marinades, dressings, and as a tangy ingredient in cooking.

How to Grow

Yarrow is a drought-resistant, resilient perennial that produces flowers from June to September. Its rigid, flattened flower heads comprise numerous minuscule blossoms, the nuclei of which may differ.

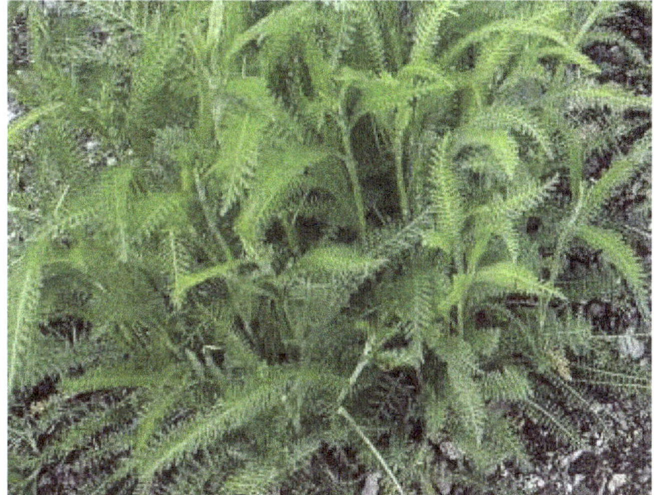

To cultivate it, select a location that receives direct sunlight.

The optimal soil is sandy and varies in quality from average to subpar. This plant has no particular preference for loam that is abundant in organic matter.

Fertilized soil is conducive to its growth; however, excessive rapidity and subsequent legginess may cause the stems to collapse when burdened with weighty flowers.

The optimal pH range for the soil is 4.0 to 8.0. A value of 6.4 is regarded as the optimal value. Make arrangements for the agricultural extension office in your area to perform a soil analysis to determine the pH of your soil.

It is possible that the drainage is exceptional, despite the moderately poor soil quality. Yarrow is not tolerant of damp feet, nor does it thrive in humid environments.

Achillea prefers arid, hot conditions. However, there are cultivated hybrid series that can tolerate some humidity, including Galaxy and Seduction.

At maturity, plants typically attain a height of two to four feet. However, certain botanical species, particularly those found in the open, may grow shorter, and certain hybrids can reach a height of five feet. The widths vary between one and three feet.

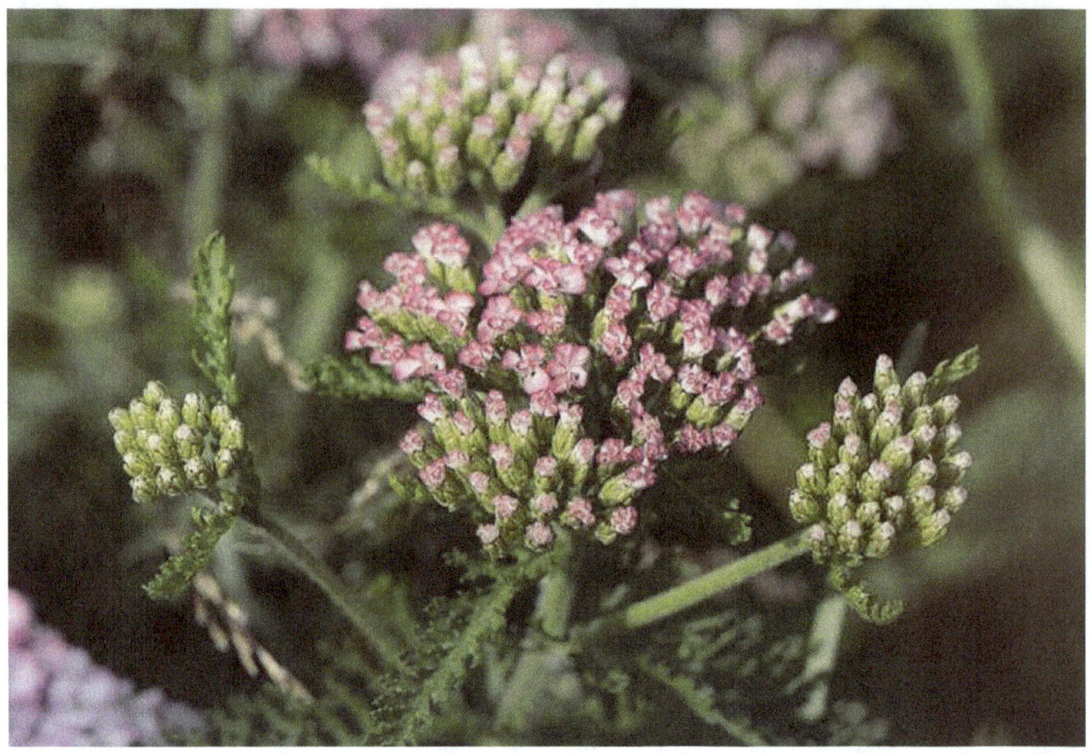

Consider mature dimensions when selecting a location for your plants. Species of Achillea exhibit robust growth patterns, attaining full maturity within the second year of development.

Regardless of whether you are starting with seeds, divisions, or tip cuttings, new plants require approximately one inch of water per week in order to develop deep, sturdy roots. If an inch of precipitation falls, additional irrigation is unnecessary.

Once established, yarrow exhibits remarkable resistance to drought and water scarcity. If a dry spell persists, however, moisten the plant instead of testing its tolerance.

Growing Tips

A robust plant such as yarrow, once established, exerts considerable effort in the garden, particularly when these three success guidelines are kept in mind:

- Choose cultivars that tolerate high levels of humidity if necessary.
- Poor soil is preferable to rich soil for encouraging the growth of compact, moderately-paced plants.
- Merely not watering does not imply drought tolerance.

Your plants will reward you with years of color in exchange for a small amount of maintenance if you give them a healthy start. Determine precisely how little is necessary.

Yarrow Care

Drought-tolerant common yarrow thrives in arid conditions, rendering it a prime candidate for xeriscaping, particularly for desert dwellers. Although yarrow is typically sold as plant seedlings, it is also simple to cultivate from seed and requires little care once established.

Simply make sure to plant it in soil that is well-drained, watering it routinely during drought conditions, but giving it ample time to fully dry out in between.

Common yarrow must be planted in an area where its proliferation is not a concern, despite the fact that it is technically invasive only in uncultivated areas. You may find common yarrow seed included in wildflower mixes that, once planted and mature, make a great option for a cutting garden.

- **Light**

Yarrow thrives in a garden bed that is exposed to direct sunlight, as this facilitates its compact growth and increases the quantity of blossoms produced. This plant can tolerate partial shade, yet inadequate sunlight may cause it to grow long and spindly, necessitating staking.

- **Soil**

Common yarrow is capable of thriving in sandy, loamy, and clay soils, among others. Regardless of the medium, this plant thrives in well-drained, dry conditions. Fertilizer and compost should be avoided whenever possible, as nutrient-rich soil promotes potentially undesirable and aggressive growth.

- **Water**

Once established, common yarrow can tolerate drought conditions. Regular, moderate irrigation will suffice to promote germination and facilitate the development of tender seedlings. Thereafter, weekly watering of only half an inch is sufficient to sustain growth.

During periods of natural precipitation, completely refrain from irrigation, particularly if the weekly water input reaches or exceeds one inch.

- **Moisture and temperature**

Yarrow flourishes in warm summer conditions (65 to 75 degrees Fahrenheit), but can begin to develop heat damage at temperatures above 86 degrees Fahrenheit. Although yarrow is typically perceived as a laid-back creature, it is adverse to chilly drafts and temperatures close to freezing.

While yarrow can tolerate a certain degree of moisture, it prefers arid conditions and is susceptible to developing root rot or fungus in saturated soil.

- **Fertilizer**

Yarrow plants require little attention in terms of nutrition. A spring side-dressing of compost on an annual basis should be sufficient for the duration of the season. Some cultivators, however, opt not to fertilize this plant at all, as nutrient-rich soil could promote invasive propagation.

How to Harvest

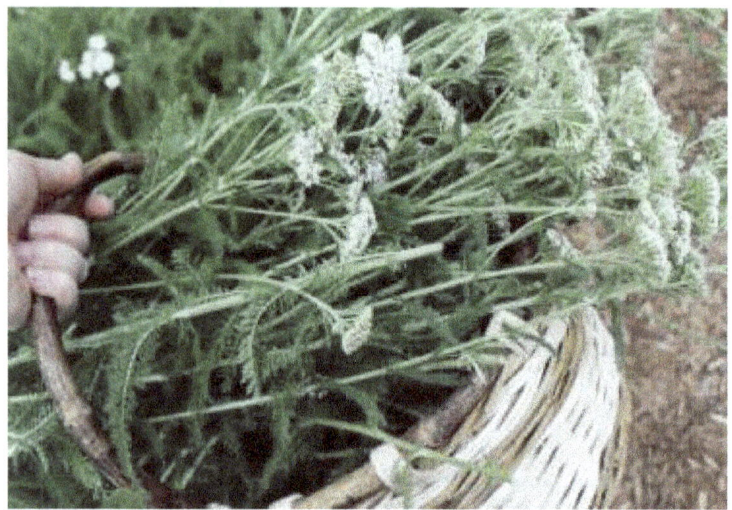

Yarrow should be harvested at its peak of blossoming throughout the summer. When harvesting, ensure that the plants appear robust and are fully or nearly fully bloomed.

Additionally, choose a sunny day after moisture has evaporated but prior to the dissipation of essential oils. To reduce the risk of developing contact dermatitis, wear gloves, and for precise incisions, utilize shears. You will want to cut the yarrow plant at the stem, about 2 inches above the earth.

Dosing

Yarrow has been utilized mainly by adults in the form of tea or plant extract. It has also been utilized in gargles and administered as an ointment or cream. Consult a healthcare professional regarding the optimal product type and dosage for a particular medical condition.

How to Dry Yarrow

To dry the plant, agitate the cut sections to remove any insects or beetles that may be present. Then, stretch out in a dry, cold, and dark location. A drying platform for herbs is ideal for this purpose. Alternatively, you could position the plants in a paper bag and leave them undisturbed for a while.

I left the leaves to dry naturally after removing them from the stems. It appeared that doing so accelerated the process.

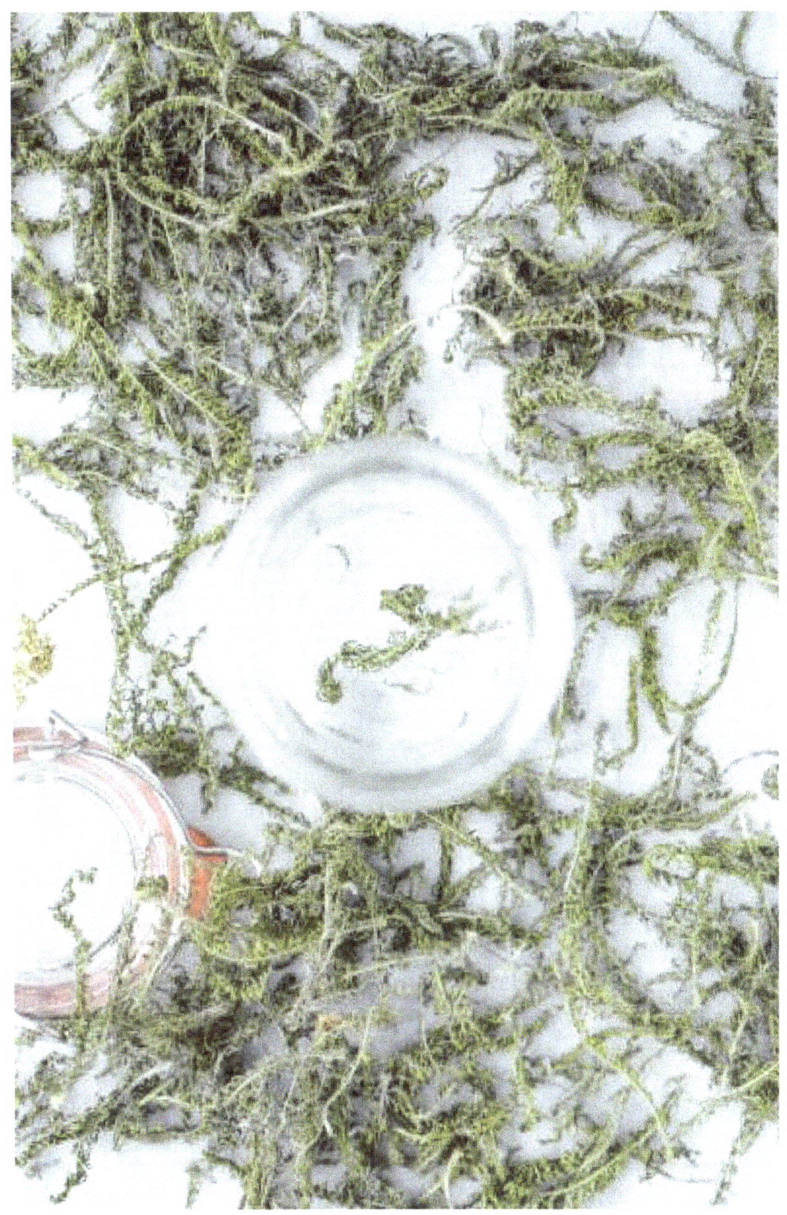

In a hurry (or if you lack the space in your home to dry herbs), you can rapidly remove the moisture by using a food dehydrator. Simply ensure that the delicate flowers and foliage are placed on the lowest setting to prevent burning.

Separate the desiccated leaves and flower tops into two airtight jars. Both jars should be labeled and stored in a cold, dark place.

CHAPTER SEVEN

PEARLY EVERLASTING

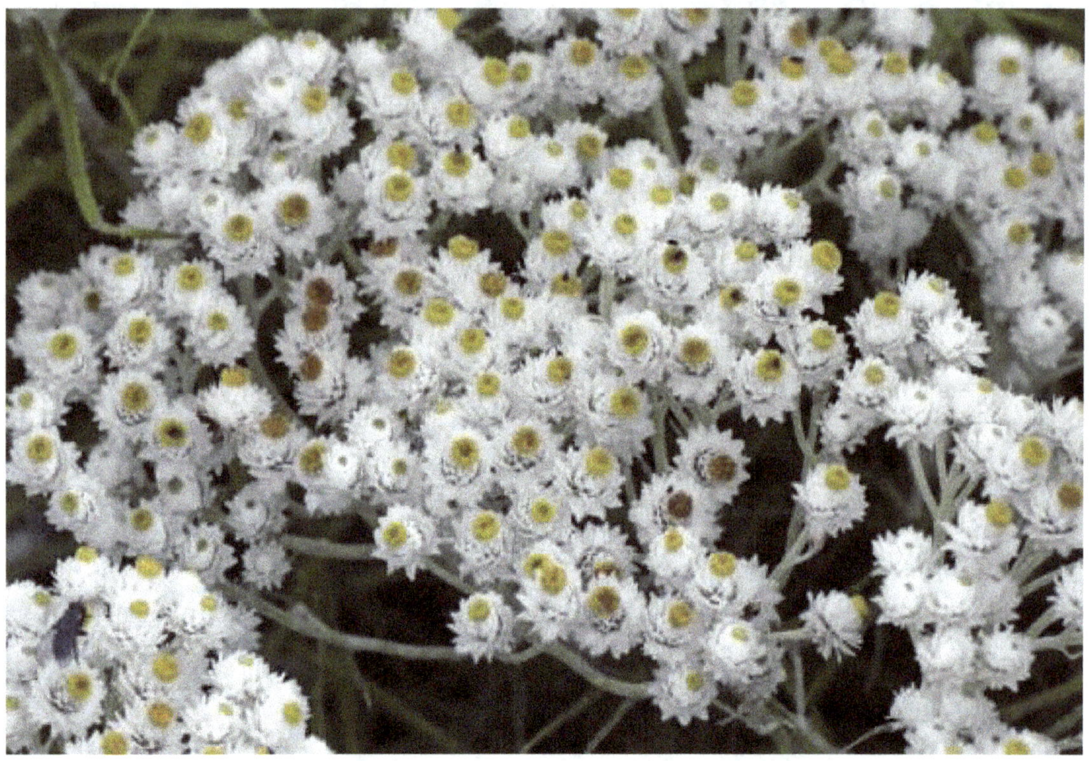

Anaphalis margaritacea, also referred to as pearly everlasting or western pearly everlasting, is a species of flowering perennial plant in the Asteraceae family that is native to Asia and North America.

Season

Pearly Everlasting tolerates frost and usually flowers in late summer, with seeds ripening in the fall.

Habitat

Pearly Everlasting thrives in arid environments such as open pastures, roadway edges, and wastelands.

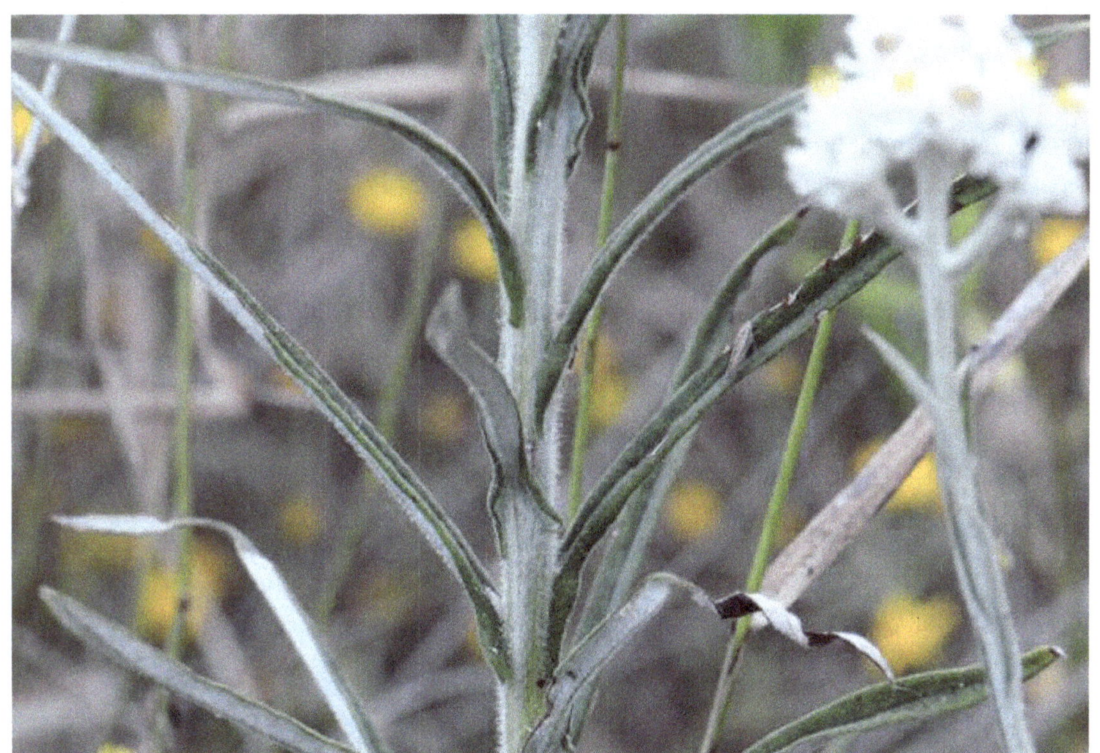

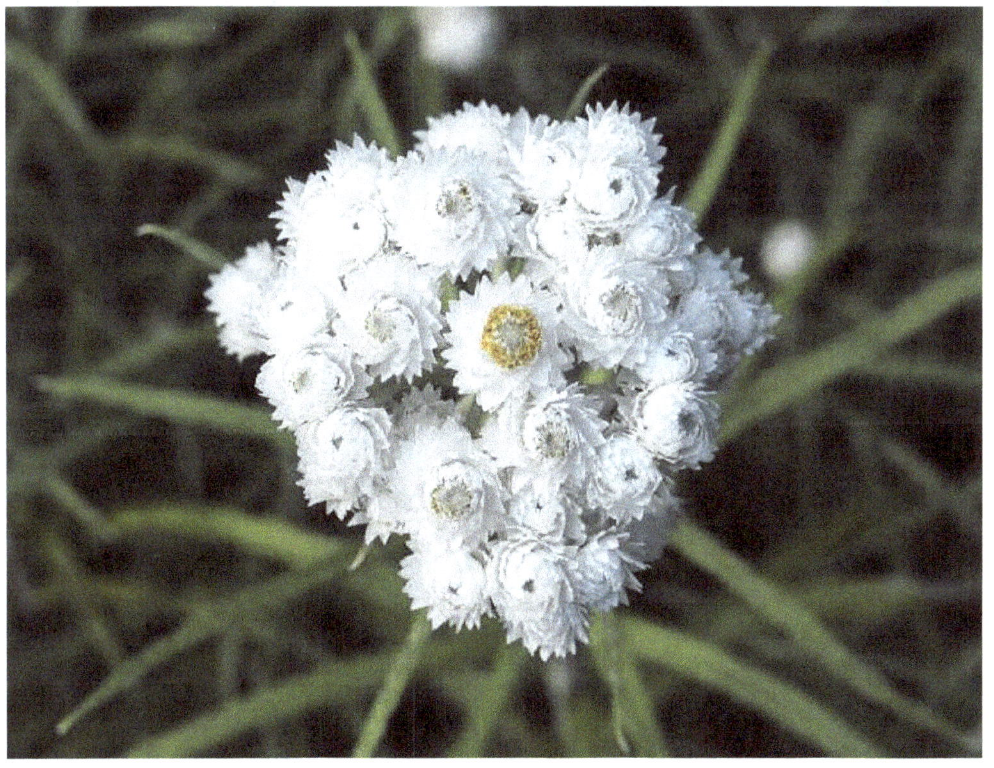

Wildflower Anaphalis maragitacea is likely one of the simplest botanicals to distinguish. Originating in North America, this species inhabits nearly the entire continent, excluding the humid southeast. When engaging in pearly, everlasting foraging, it is prudent to take into account the following distinguishing characteristics:

- Tends to grow at higher elevations
- Like rocky, even disturbed soils
- Tolerant of both moderate shade and full sun; extremely adaptable
- Is tolerant of cool environments, including coastal highlands
- Often seen along mountain roadways or in clear cuts
- Lance-shaped, slender, woolly stems and foliage that are a tranquil grey-green hue with a paler, downy underside
- Under specific conditions, the alternately arranged leaves on a stem can reach a maximum height of 3 feet (in the Pacific Northwest, plants typically range in height from 18 to 24 feet).
- The flowers and foliage exude a mildly sweet, woodsy scent.
- In early summer, pearlescent white flower blooms emerge; as the flower matures, bracts resembling petals unveil a yellow-orange core that is distinctive of numerous plants in the Asteraceae family.

Harvest pearly everlasting in mid-summer, prior to the complete maturation of the blossom buds. The herb dries exceptionally well, retaining a substantial amount of its color and aroma. Dry pearly everlasting in a jar or container with a tight-fitting closure and store in a cool location out of direct sunlight Additionally, desiccated pearly everlasting can be tinctured for use in oil infusions.

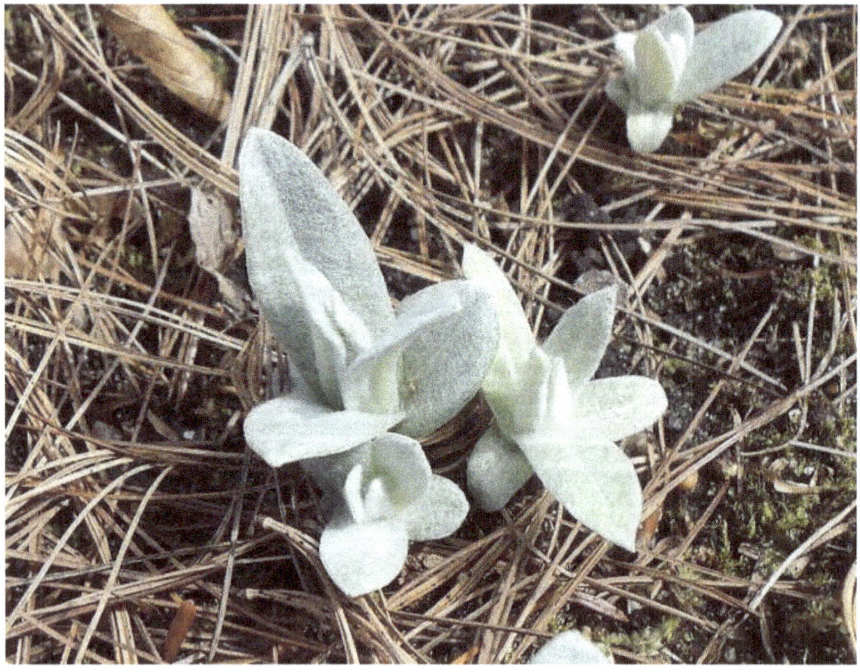

Medicinal Uses of Pearly Everlasting

Pearly Everlasting, being an indigenous plant of North America, has a substantial historical record of utilization by indigenous populations and early colonizers.

It surprises me that this herb, which provides numerous benefits, is underutilized in domestic apothecaries. When the first sign of sinus obstruction from an impending cold appears in early autumn, I frequently recall the word pearly.

Additionally, in spring, when seasonal allergies cause sinuses to become full and drippy, I recall the word pearly. Pearly Everlasting, when consumed as a tea or vapor, aids in the clearance of the respiratory tract and the cessation of excessive mucus secretion. It is also a suitable herbal remedy for a persistent throat tickle and irritation accompanied by a moist, chesty cough.

When a low-grade fever and mild shivers persist, a steamy bath or sauna filled with a lot of pearly will encourage perspiration and make it easier to get rid of the pain and discomfort that come with the flu and colds.

As an alternative to tobacco, pearly everlasting was also utilized as a medicinal smoke to treat respiratory ailments such as pneumonia and bronchitis.

An additional conventional application of Anaphalis margaritacea is to alleviate rigid rheumatic joints. When this herb is exposed to moist heat, such as through the use of a poultice or herbal vapor, it has been linked to enhanced range of motion. The combination of this anti-inflammatory effect and reduced joint rigidity may hold great promise for individuals suffering from rheumatoid arthritis.

Additionally, pearly everlasting is highly compatible with the digestive system. This herb's cooling and astringent properties render it suitable for the treatment of excessive gastric mucus that induces frequent coughing and throat clearing, ulcer conditions accompanied by elevated body temperature, food poisoning, diarrhea, and ulcers.

A further traditional application of pearly everlasting is as a form of care for one's deceased. Pearly, being an astringent antiseptic, promotes expeditious wound closure and thoroughly clean recovery. Additionally, it reduces the size of boils and blisters and accelerates their recuperation when applied to these areas.

Uses for Pearly Everlasting

Home herbalists had previously employed pearly everlasting as a:

- Herbal infusion or beverage
- Medicinal vapor

- Herbal smoke
- Herbal poultice or adhesive
- The process of fermentation
- Tincture
- Tub or sauna immersion
- Infused vegetable oil

How to Grow

In the early spring, prior to the last frost, it is optimal to distribute Anaphalis directly onto the soil surface and then lightly dust the soil around it with a spacing of 20 to 30 cm.

Pearly everlastings are tolerant of arid conditions and prefer either partially shady or full sunlight. It is essential that the soil be well-drained.

Ten to seventy days are necessary for anaphalis to germinate. When propagating pearly everlasting from seed indoors, the optimal germination temperature range is 13 to 18 degrees Celsius.

Seven weeks should pass before transferring them to the outdoor environment in late spring, following the final chill.

Caring for Pearly Everlasting

Regarding maintenance, pearly everlasting is remarkably self-sufficient; all that is required is sunlight. It thrives in regions that receive partial to full sunlight, exhibits drought tolerance, and requires minimal fertilization or other soil amendments.

Dosage, Safety, and Precautions

Pearly, similar to numerous indigenous and traditional botanicals, lacks comprehensive guidelines regarding safety and dosage. Herbalists generally regard it as a safe botanical; however, as with any novel substance, exercise prudence when utilizing it.

As Anaphalis margaritacea may inhibit milk production, lactating mothers should avoid using it. Prior to using this herb or any other, individuals who are pregnant, taking prescription medications, or have a chronic illness should seek the advice of a physician.

How to Store

When the flower centers develop a dark brown hue, the seeds of Pearly Everlasting have reached maturity. Detach the heads and disperse them in an area shielded from direct sunlight to dry. In order to extract the seed material from the papery husk, thresh the heads. In a cold, dry location, store Pearly Everlasting seeds.

CHAPTER EIGHT

OREGON GRAPE

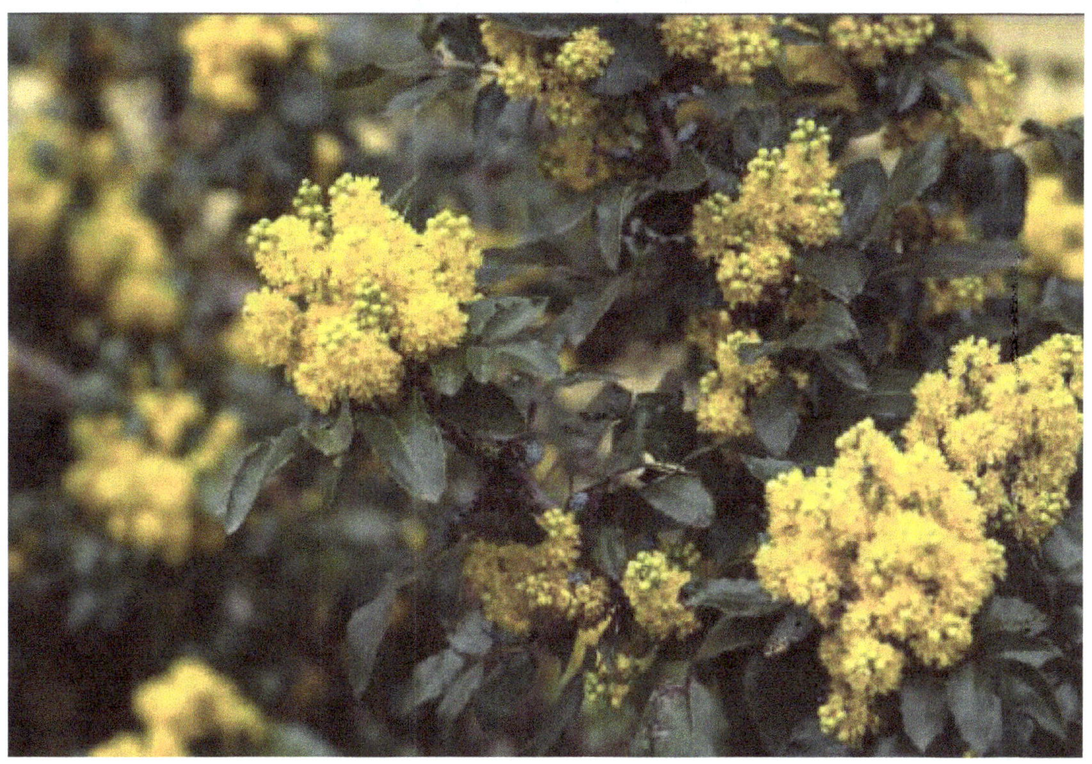

A species of flowering plant belonging to the Berberidaceae family, Berberis aquifolium is indigenous to western North America and is also known as the Oregon grape or holly-leaved barberry.

Pinnate leaves comprised of spiny leaflets adorn its 1–3 meter (3–10 foot) in height and 1.5 meter (5 ft) in width. In early spring, it produces dense clusters of yellow blossoms, which are followed by berries that are dark bluish-black in color.

Certain indigenous peoples of the Pacific Northwest consume the blossoms, and the species is officially designated as the state flower of Oregon.

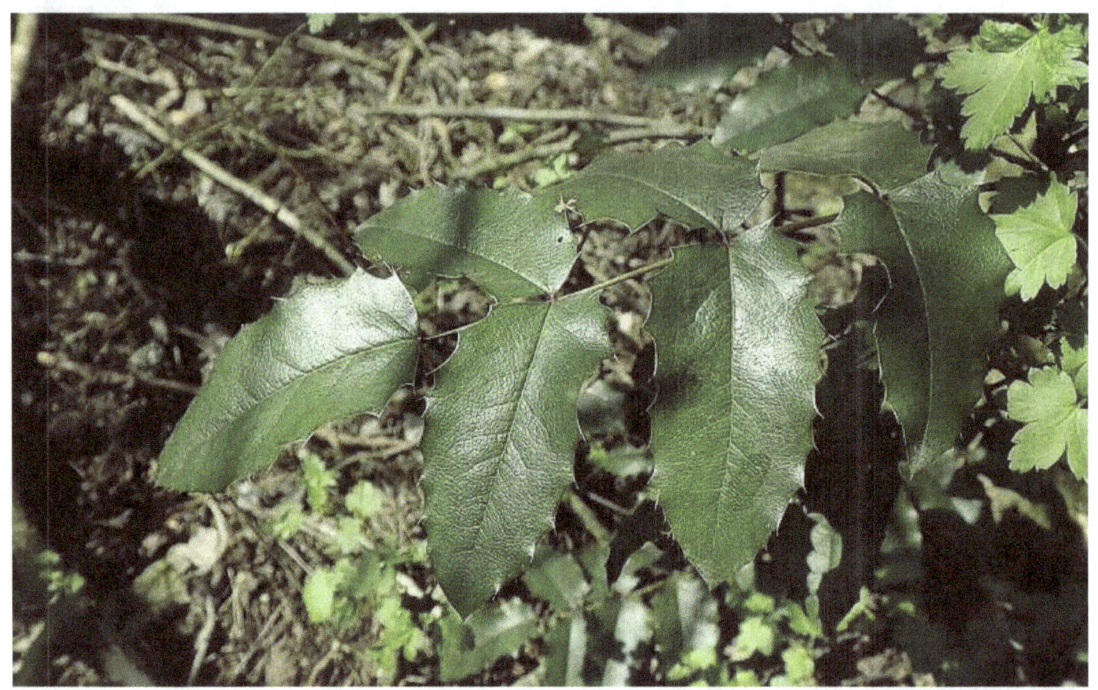

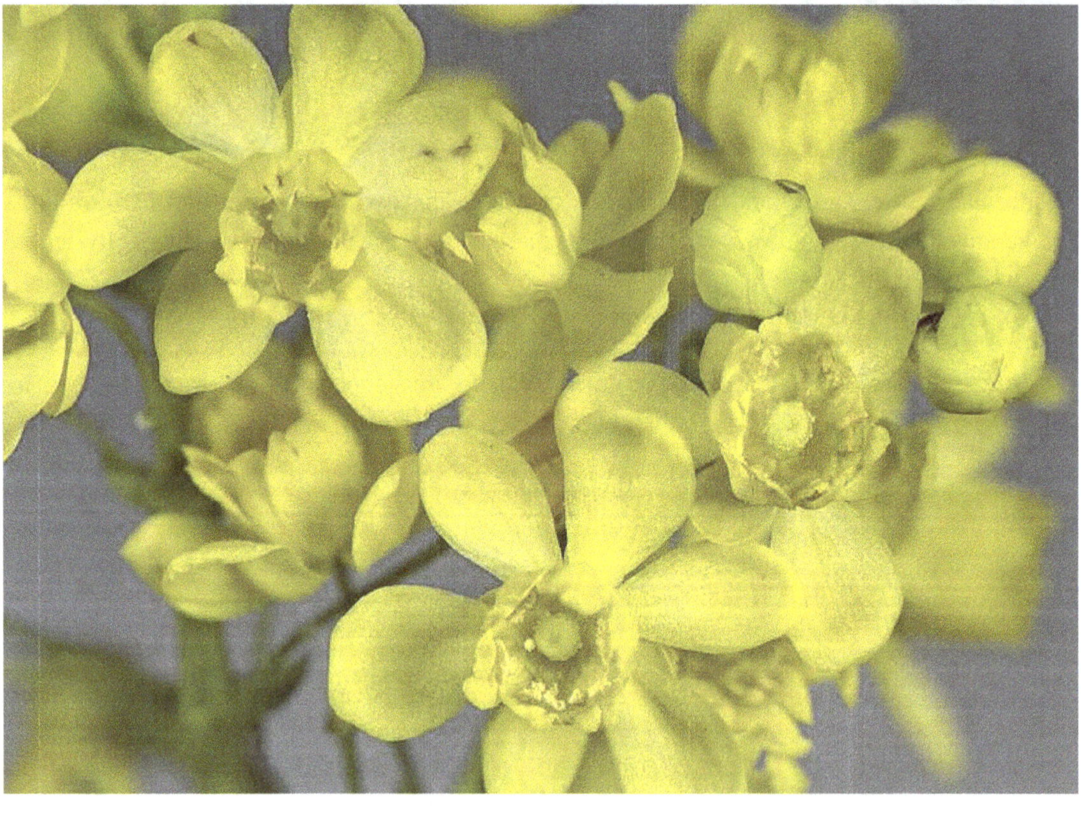

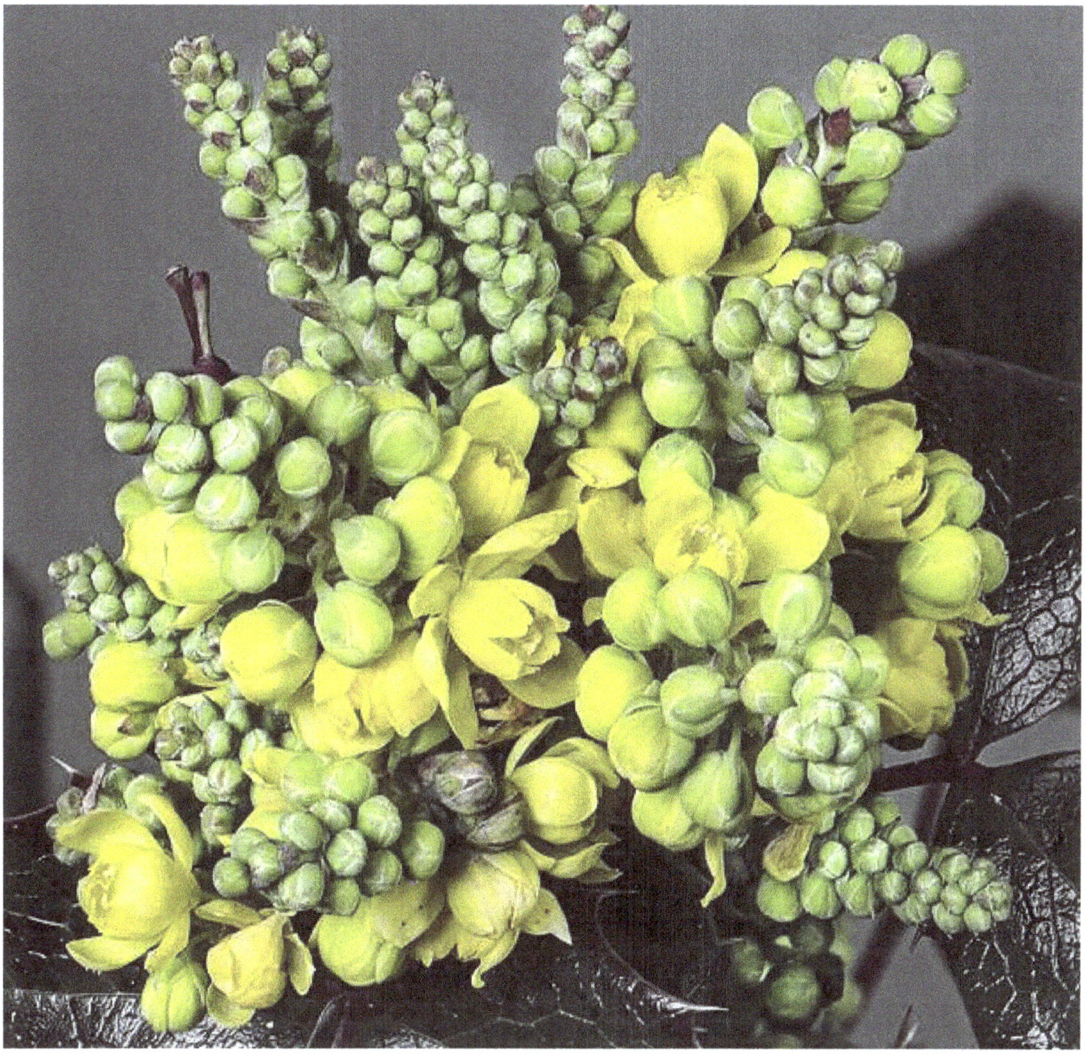

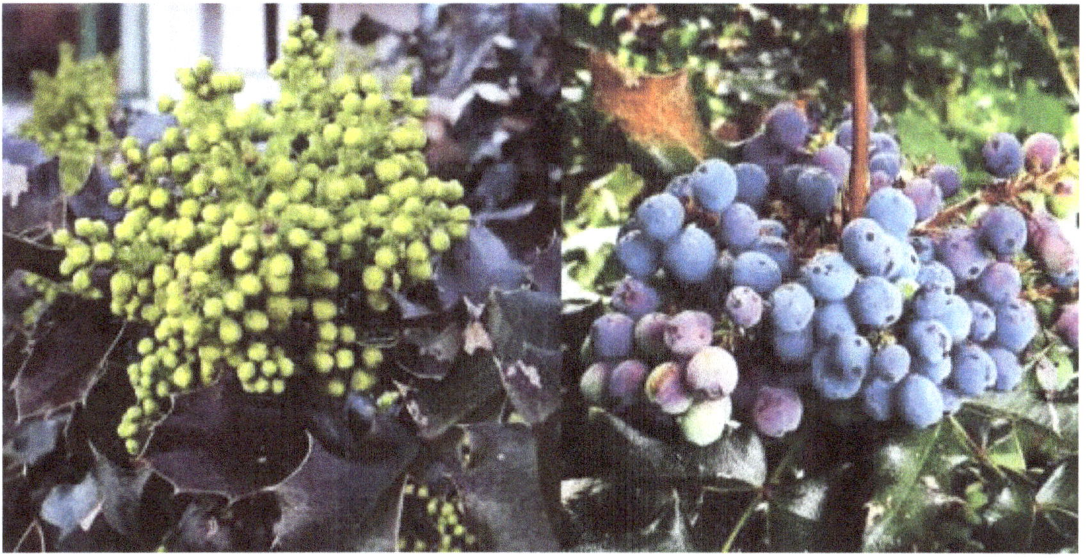

- **Growth**

The Oregon Grape, which attains a height of 6–8 feet (2–2.5 m), extends its underground stems to a width of approximately 5 feet (1.5m). It may initially develop a sluggish growth rate as it becomes established, but it will mature rapidly.

- **Leaves**

Shiny with sharp spikes, looking just like a holly leaf

- **Flowers**

Small, brilliant yellow blossoms droop in clusters above the foliage during the spring, summer, fall, and winter.

- **Fruit**

Prolonged assemblages of violet to black fruit are enveloped in a delicate blossom that imparts a blue hue.

- **Stem**

Woody

- **Taste**

When combined with other sweet berries or sweeteners, such as honey or sugar, the naturally sour berries become a delectable treat.

Season

The optimal time to harvest Oregon grape roots is in late autumn or winter, subsequent to seed formation.

Habitat

Mostly in gardens and parks but occasionally spreading to the wild, as this picture of Mahonia in woodland shows

Medicinal Uses

In addition to its edible fruit, the Oregon grape is widely recognized for its medicinal properties. It is predominantly composed of the compound berberine, which is discovered in the plant's roots and bark. Berberine has properties that are antibiotic, antimicrobial, antiviral, and antifungal.

Goldenseal root, which also contains the primary medicinal compound berberine, and Oregon grape root have comparable potential applications.

In the low wild variety, berberine is essentially only present in the roots; however, in the tall variety, the stems are considerably larger, allowing access to it through the shaving of the bark. It possesses a distinct yellow color.

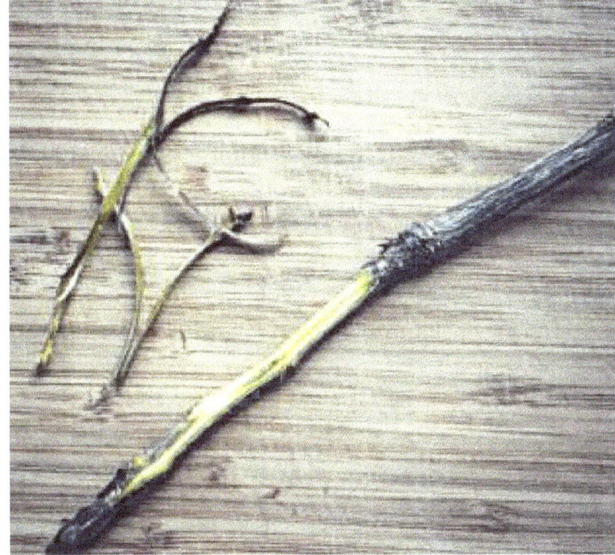

The stems and roots may be utilized to create a salve, tincture, oil infusion, or tea. However, for the time being, I will contemplate what to do with these magnificent berries!

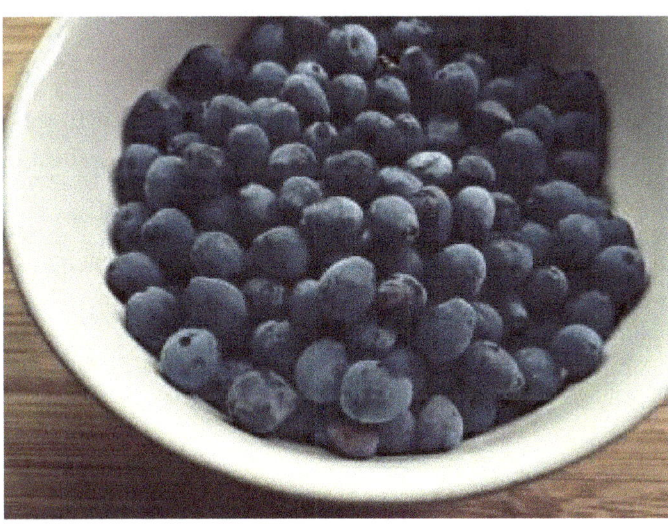

From where these originated, there is much more, and I'm considering a possible collaboration. I am also intrigued by the possibility of experimenting with a salve made from the roots and stems of infusions of tea or oil.

Potential Uses

The Oregon grape is a multipurpose plant that possesses a multitude of additional potential advantages.

- **Antibacterial properties are possible.**

Berberine, an antimicrobial compound found in Oregon grapes, exhibits potent properties. Primarily, it is employed to treat bacterial parasitic infections and diarrhea.

Additionally, Oregon grape extracts have been shown to possess antimicrobial activity against specific pathogenic bacteria, fungi, and protozoa, according to a test-tube investigation.

Numerous studies have yielded comparable findings, suggesting that berberine has the potential to combat bacterial infections, including those caused by E. coli and MRSA.

- **May relieve several stomach issues**

The Oregon grape contains berberine, which may alleviate the symptoms of irritable bowel syndrome (IBS) and other stomach conditions such as inflammation of the intestines.

Compared to those who received a placebo, those who received berberine in an 8-week study involving 196 individuals with IBS reported reductions in diarrhea frequency, abdominal pain, and overall IBS symptoms

Animal studies employing this compound have demonstrated potential ameliorations in various gastric ailments, including gastrointestinal inflammation, in addition to symptoms associated with IBS.

However, research on the effects of the Oregon grape on gastrointestinal inflammation in humans is still scarce.

- **May help ease heartburn**

By virtue of berberine's anti-inflammatory properties, the Oregon grape may aid in the prevention of heartburn and associated esophageal injury.

Acid reflux means that gastric acid ascends into the esophagus, causing heartburn to be a frequent symptom. Heartburn is characterized by a burning, excruciating ache in the chest or throat.

In a study involving rodents with acid reflux, omeprazole, a common pharmaceutical treatment for heartburn, caused more esophageal damage than berberine.

Remember that human research is absolutely necessary.

- **May help improve your mood**

There is some evidence to suggest that berberine, an active compound found in Oregon grapes, might mitigate symptoms associated with chronic stress and depression.

A 15-day study on rodents revealed that dopamine and serotonin levels increased by 52% and 19%, respectively, in response to berberine treatment.

These hormones are recognized for their role in mood regulation.

However, further investigation on humans is required prior to recommending the Oregon grape as a potential treatment for depression.

How to Grow Oregon Grapes

Mahonia aquifolium, the state flower of Oregon, grows into a magnificent ornamental shrub that provides visual appeal throughout all four seasons. While it can tolerate both full sun and full shade (although intense heat and sunlight reflected off solid surfaces may cause leaf scorching), it prefers dappled or partial shade to flourish.

The Oregon grape prefers well-drained, slightly acidic soils that are abundant in hummus. It thrives in similar environmental conditions as rhododendrons, azaleas, salal, huckleberry, and blueberries; in fact, it is frequently observed coexisting with these plants in its natural habitat.

The holly-like foliage of Oregon grapes begins as crimson-colored new growth, matures to a vibrant emerald green, and in the fall and winter, it blushes burgundy bronze. Thus, to put it another way, this "evergreen" is not merely green. Bright yellow blossoms attract pollinators to the garden in the spring.

When the grape-shaped fruits, which develop a dark blue hue and a distinct "microbial bloom," succumb to light to moderate pressure in mid- to late summer, they are ripe.

In addition to its aesthetic appeal, the Oregon grape contributes to the overall value of the landscape through its role as a shrub. Security is that value. Situated beneath windows that provide access while maintaining privacy, the prickly foliage is certain to thwart even the most audacious intruders.

In native landscapes, one may also encounter low-growing, trailing varieties of Oregon grape (Mahonia repens).

How to Care

The Oregon Grape is an extremely uncommon houseplant that requires consistent watering and is simple to cultivate. They thrive in direct sunlight and should be positioned no closer than three feet from a window. Oregon grapes prefer well-draining soil.

How to Harvest

When seeds have formed, in late autumn or winter, Oregon grape roots are at their peak. To harvest, elevate the plant from the soil using force from the base of the stem and remove a portion of the root that is liftable.

Brush away any debris and soil with care so as not to cause injury to the outer root bark.

Preserve stems for a minimum of three feet.

CHAPTER NINE

GOLDENROD

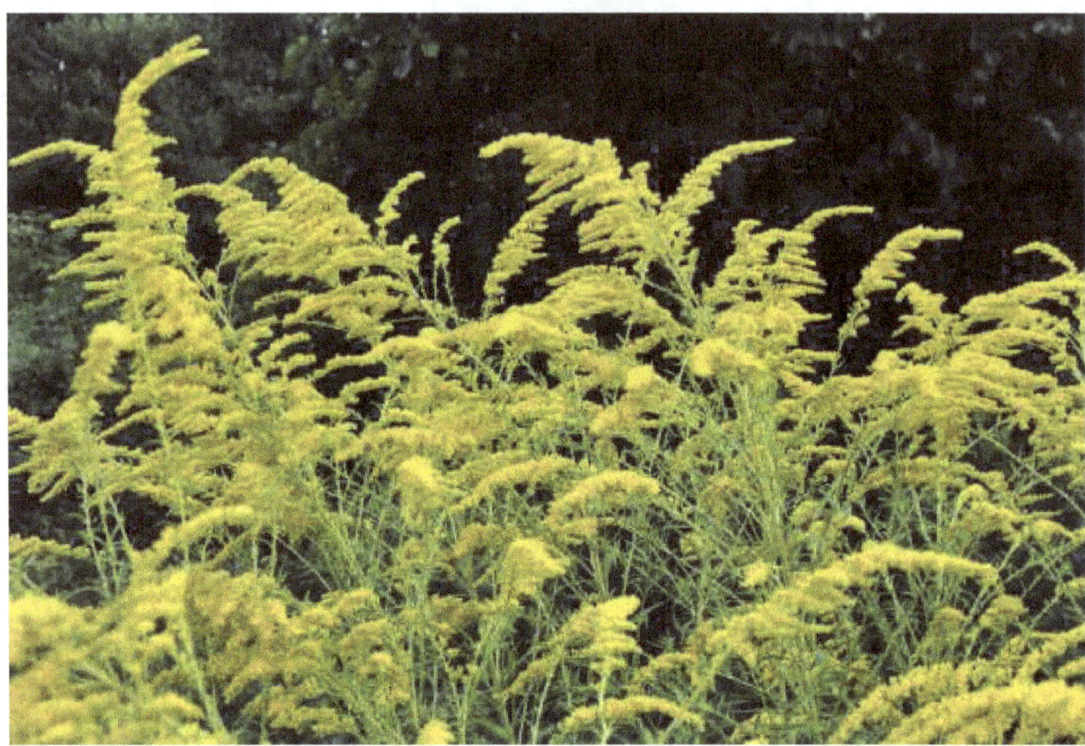

Asteraceae, a weedy, typically perennial herbaceous genus comprising approximately 150 species, includes goldenrod (genus Solidago). While the majorities are indigenous to North America, a limited number of species flourish in Europe and Asia. Goldenrods are a distinctive flora of eastern North America, where an estimated sixty species are found. They are prevalent across nearly all habitat types, including woodlands, marshes, mountains, fields, and roadside areas, and are among the most magnificent autumn flowers from the Great Plains to the Atlantic.

Identification

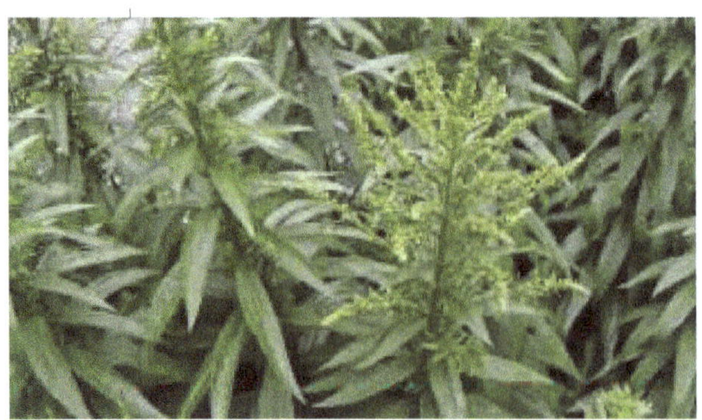

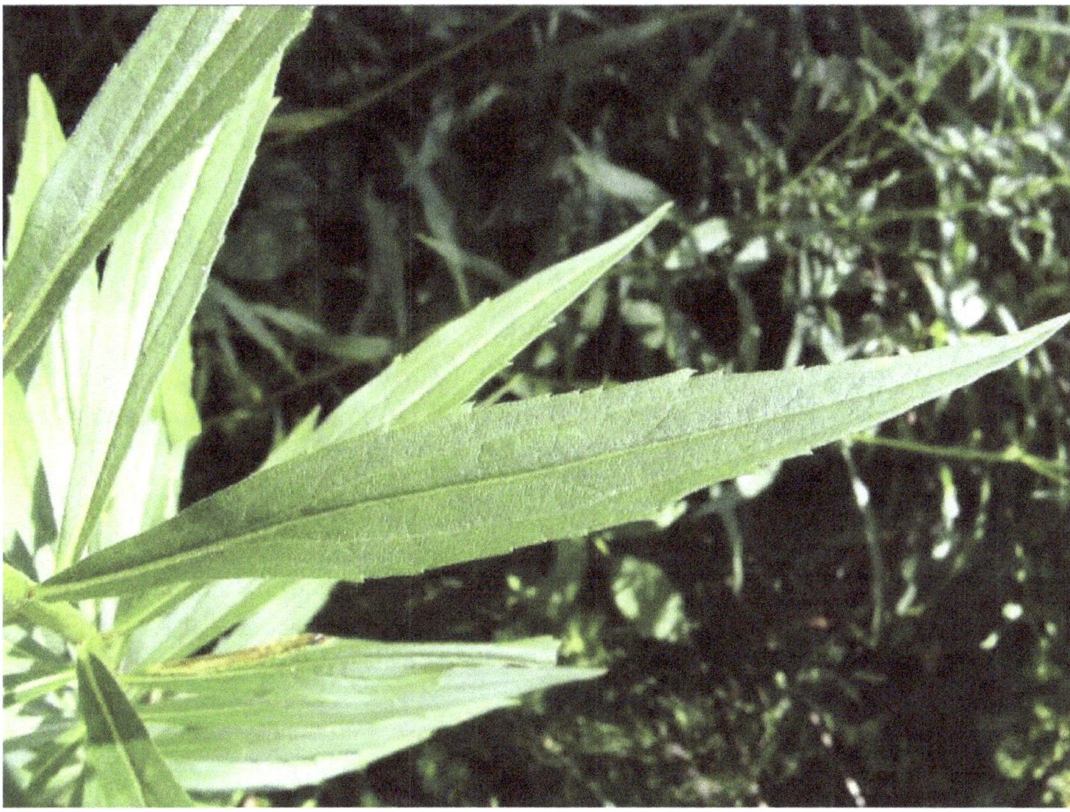

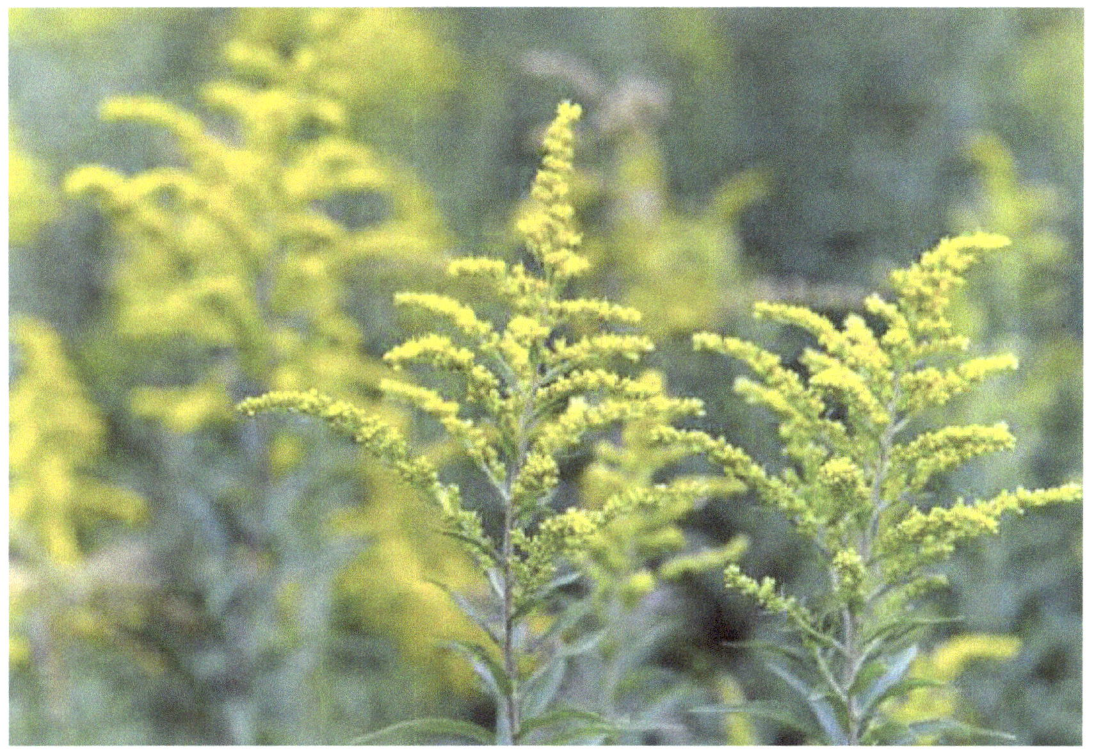

- **Distinguishing Features**

Prolonged, woody stems adorned with spiky, tooth-like structures support dense clusters of yellow, widely dispersed flowers.

- **Flowers**

Goldenrod flowers develop in a broad or, at times, narrow pyramidal panicle as an inflorescence. Varying in height from 5 to 40 cm (2 to 16 inches), they are virtually the same width.

The upper surfaces of the numerous to numerous horizontal branches are adorned with a profusion of small, densely clustered heads of golden yellow flowers. The length and width of each individual flower head are approximately 3 mm (1/8"). Flowers appear on this plant from mid-July to September.

- **Leaves**

Goldenrod leaves are approximately 10 centimeters in length and 2 centimeters in width, tapering to a point at the apex and narrowing at the base; they lack a leaf stem and have minute fangs along the periphery.

Three veins emanate in a parallel line from the leaf's base. Particularly along the veins, the underside of the leaf is hairy, whereas the upper surface has a rough texture.

- **Height**

A typical plant measures one meter in height.

- **Edible Parts**

Every aerial component of the plant is edible. The blossoms are edible and embellish salads with aesthetic appeal. To prepare tea, fresh or dried flowers and foliage are utilized. In addition to being cooked like spinach and incorporated into casseroles, stews, and soups, leaves can be blanched and preserved for use in stir-fry, stews, or soups during the winter and spring.

Season

From late summer through mid-fall

Habitat

September and October are goldenrod months with an abundance of supplies. This yellow plant is found in orchards, forests, fields, roadsides, compost mounds, and moist environments in Canada.

<u>*Benefits and Medicinal Uses of Goldenrod*</u>

- **Plants of goldenrod contribute to antioxidants.**

Goldenrod possesses a high concentration of antioxidants. Goldenrod is a valuable source of flavonoids, which are plant compounds such as quercetin and kaempferol, and is more antioxidant-rich than green tea.

- **Goldenrod benefits research: Metabolism, skin protection, cancer, and more**

Similar to numerous other plants abundant in polyphenols, goldenrod is currently undergoing research to identify potential applications in the field of medicine. Among the areas of investigation are the potential anti-obesity and anti-cancer properties of goldenrod, in addition to its ability to prevent skin degeneration.

According to some research, goldenrod might have a beneficial effect on lipids.

<u>*Traditional Goldenrod Medicinal Uses*</u>

- Herbalists hold goldenrod in high regard as a natural remedy for allergic reactions.
- Goldenrod has long been recognized as a traditional remedy for urinary tract infections and renal support due to its antimicrobial and diuretic properties. Goldenrod was approved by the European Commission for the prevention and treatment of kidney stones.
- James Duke mentions the antifungal properties of goldenrod and suggests using goldenrod tea to treat candida.
- Considered particularly beneficial for respiratory infections, goldenrod aids in the drainage of mucous and the soothing of inflamed tissues. Investigate a variety of botanicals for colds and ailments when you are experiencing a sense of malaise.
- A topical application of goldenrod facilitates skin healing.
- An oil infused with goldenrod has demonstrated potential as a topical analgesic.
- Goldenrod has the potential to alleviate inflammation within the digestive tract. Goldenrod, an astringent herb, aids in the toning of tissues.
- As a lymphatic herb, goldenrod is occasionally prescribed for arthritis and gout and is regarded as a detoxifying agent.

Native Americans have historically utilized goldenrod for its medicinal properties, among numerous others. If the notion of gathering medicinal plants captivates you, contemplate investigating dozens of additional wild herbs that are likely to be flourishing in your vicinity.

Goldenrod is an outstanding natural dye option for those who enjoy experimenting with vibrant yellow hues.

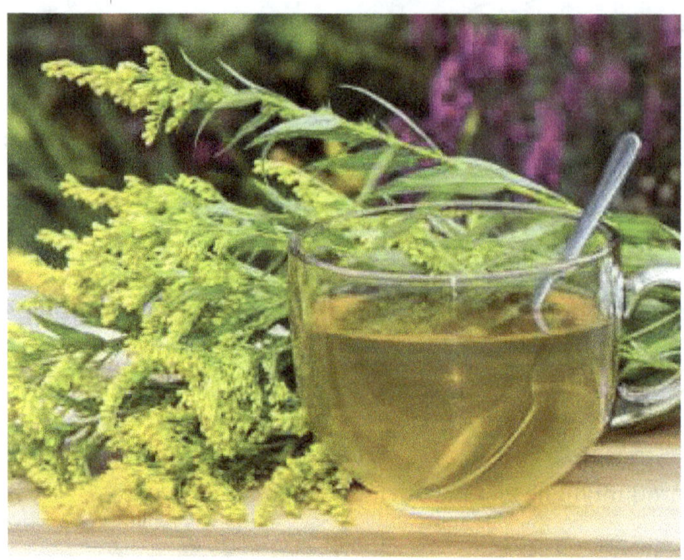

Goldenrod Tea

As expected, the flavor of goldenrod tea differs depending on the cultivar and environmental conditions. In the majority of North America, goldenrod is typically found as Solidago canadensis; however, Solidago odora is the variety most frequently used to flavor tea.

If you intend to use your goldenrod to make tea, dehydrating will enhance its flavor. If the flavor of the goldenrod plants you have access to for tea is not to your liking, I strongly suggest blending them with other herbs like lemon balm, chamomile, or mint.

- **Goldenrod Tincture**

Alternately, you could create a goldenrod tincture, in which case the flavor will be less significant.

- **Infused Oil**

A dried goldenrod plant can be used to create an infused oil for external application, either alone or in a homemade remedy.

Cautions Using Goldenrod Plant

Goldenrod handling may cause a cutaneous reaction in certain individuals. Goldenrod is a member of the aster family; therefore, individuals who have a documented allergy to asters (e.g., ragweed, daisy, or chamomile) ought to refrain from using it. Similar to other botanicals, goldenrod's safety during pregnancy has not been established. Consult your physician prior to taking goldenrod if you are currently pregnant or nursing.

Growing Goldenrod

It is simple to grow and plant goldenrod, as this plant can endure almost any environment; however, it does prefer to be cultivated in direct sunlight. Additionally, goldenrod is tolerant of a wide range of soil types that properly drain.

Goldenrod requires little maintenance once it has become established in a landscape, as the plants regrow annually. They are drought-tolerant and will require minimal, if any, irrigation. The division of clumps is required every four to five years.

Additionally, springtime cuttings may be incorporated into a garden. Mastering the cultivation of goldenrod presents numerous benefits. Insects that produce their offspring on the plant may consume pest insects that are attracted to it. Goldenrod is an attractive plant that attracts butterflies to a landscape.

Caring for Goldenrod

Goldenrod is a low-maintenance plant that requires neither watering nor nourishment. Rainfall should provide it with all the water it requires. If necessary, divide plants every three to four years; if you do not want them to self-sow, remove the deadhead. Reduce after the flowering period.

Harvesting Goldenrod

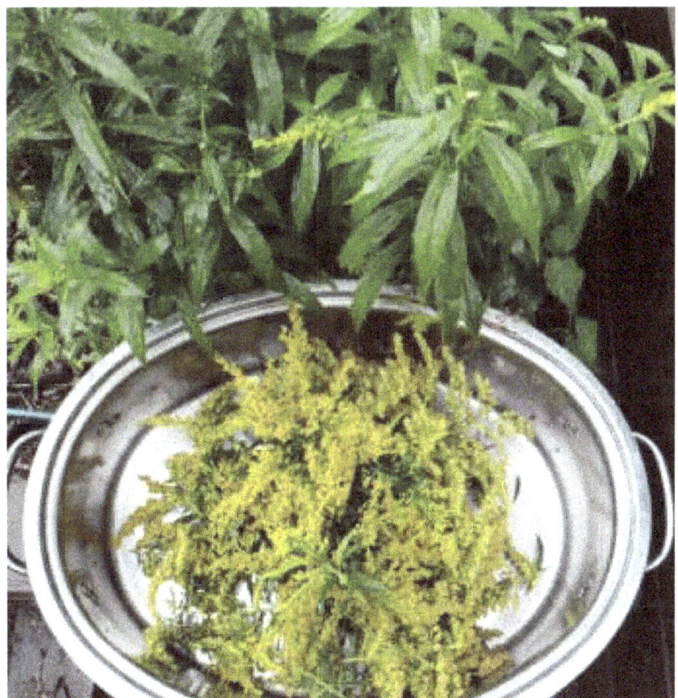

Harvest this abundant herb as soon as you notice the goldenrod's eye-catching yellow blossoms. Prepare your shears. It is generally recommended by herbalists to harvest goldenrod when the flowers are not completely exposed.

Goldenrod flowers and leaves should be in balance, so the upper half of the plant should be pruned.

Ensure that the areas from which you collect goldenrod have not been treated with herbicides. Roadsides are frequently sprayed; therefore, caution should be exercised when harvesting from roadside areas.

Dosage and form

Goldenrod is available in the following forms: botanical tea, liquid extracts, and pills.

To facilitate dosing, liquid extracts are packaged in vessels equipped with droppers. Blends containing dried extracts of goldenrod, such as juniper berry, are more frequently encountered in the form of capsules and tablets.

Dosages have not yet been thoroughly evaluated in human investigations; however, conventional medicine doses indicate the following:

- **Tea**

0.5 grams (1.2 teaspoons) of powdered goldenrod per 237 milliliters (1 cup) of boiled water

After allowing it to settle for 10–15 minutes under cover, strain. No more than four times per day.

- **Liquid extract**

Up to 0.2–0.3 ml three times daily

- **Dry extract**

Up to 350–450 mg, three times daily

These dosage recommendations are for adults and adolescents. Goldenrod is typically contraindicated for children younger than 12 years old on account of insufficient safety data.

Typically, goldenrod is applied to a particular malady for a duration of two to four weeks.

Drying Goldenrod

Drying goldenrod, similar to numerous other herbs, involves simply tying bundles together and suspending them inverted. Goldenrod flowers and foliage should become brittle and crumbly within a week in arid climates.

When desiccated, goldenrod flowers that were harvested when they were completely open may become slightly airy; however, their medicinal value remains unaffected.

Once completely dehydrated, place the dried flowers and foliage of goldenrod in an airtight container.

CHAPTER TEN

JUNIPER

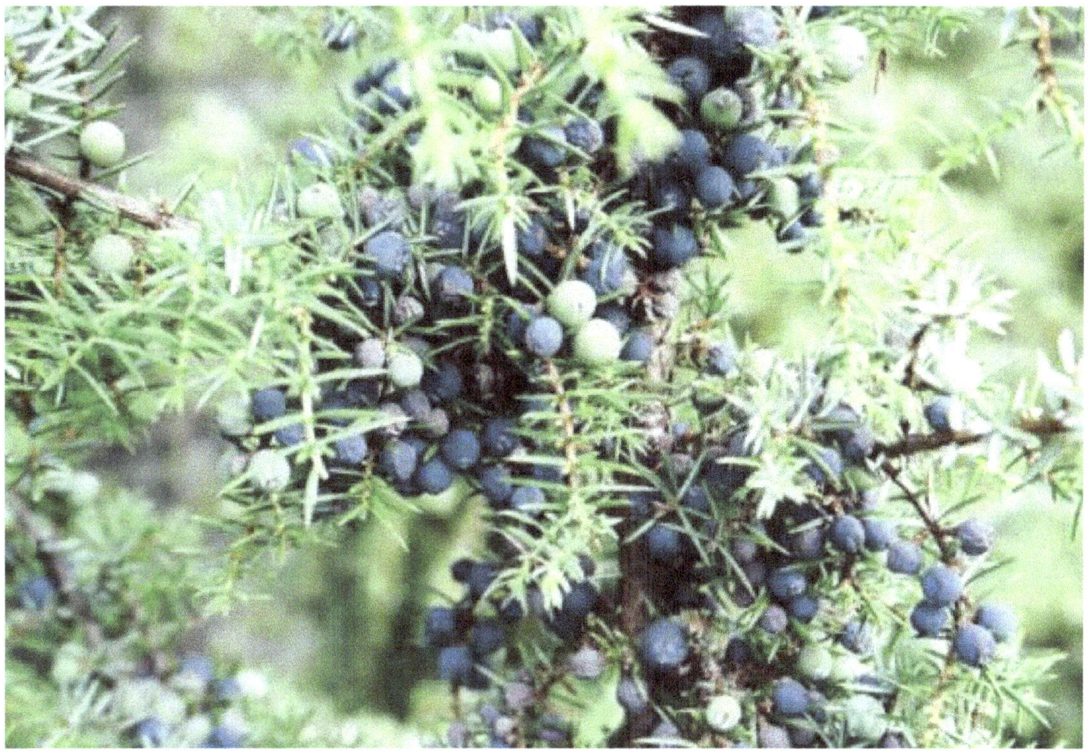

The common juniper (Juniperus communis) is a species of diminutive tree or shrub belonging to the Cupressaceae family of cypresses. Consisting of evergreen conifers, this particular plant possesses the most extensive circumpolar distribution of any woody plant in the temperate and chilly Northern Hemisphere.

Identification

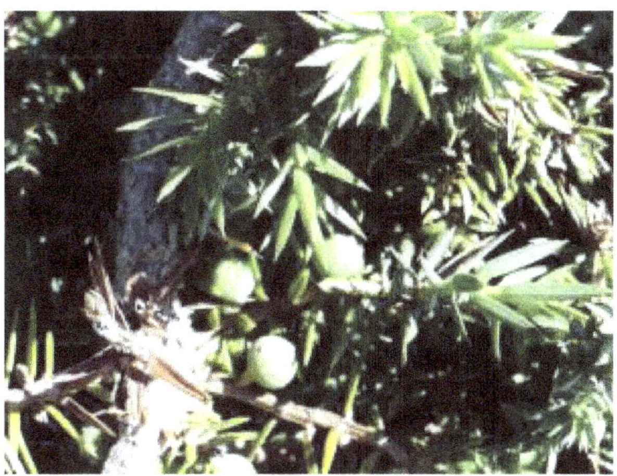

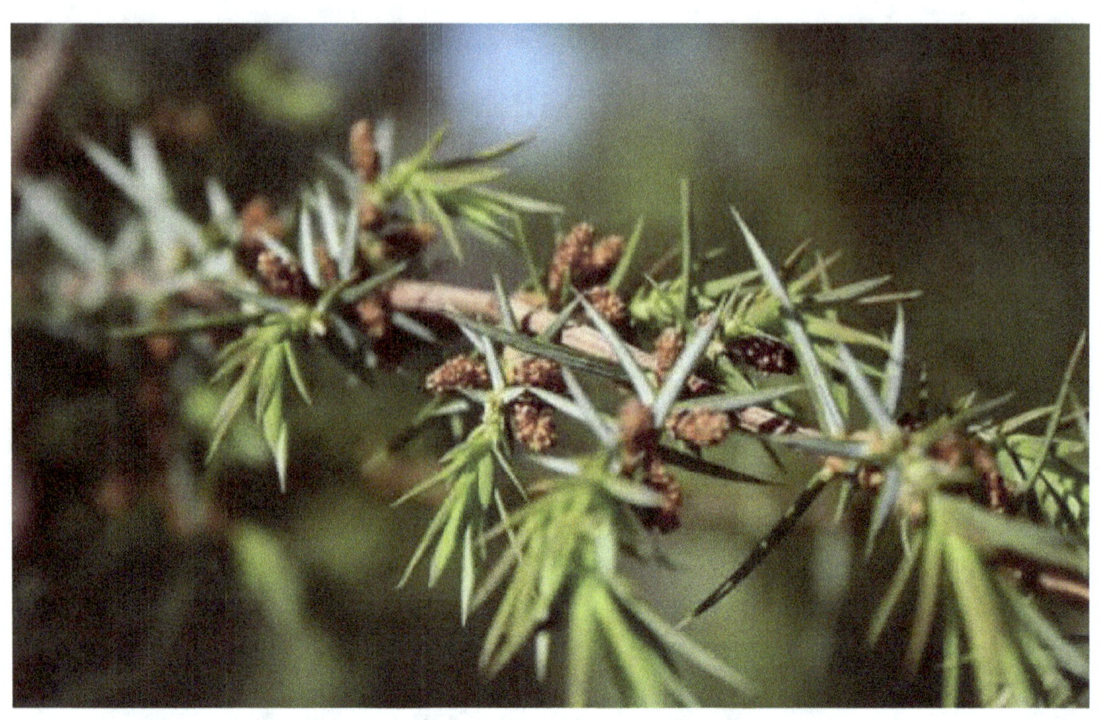

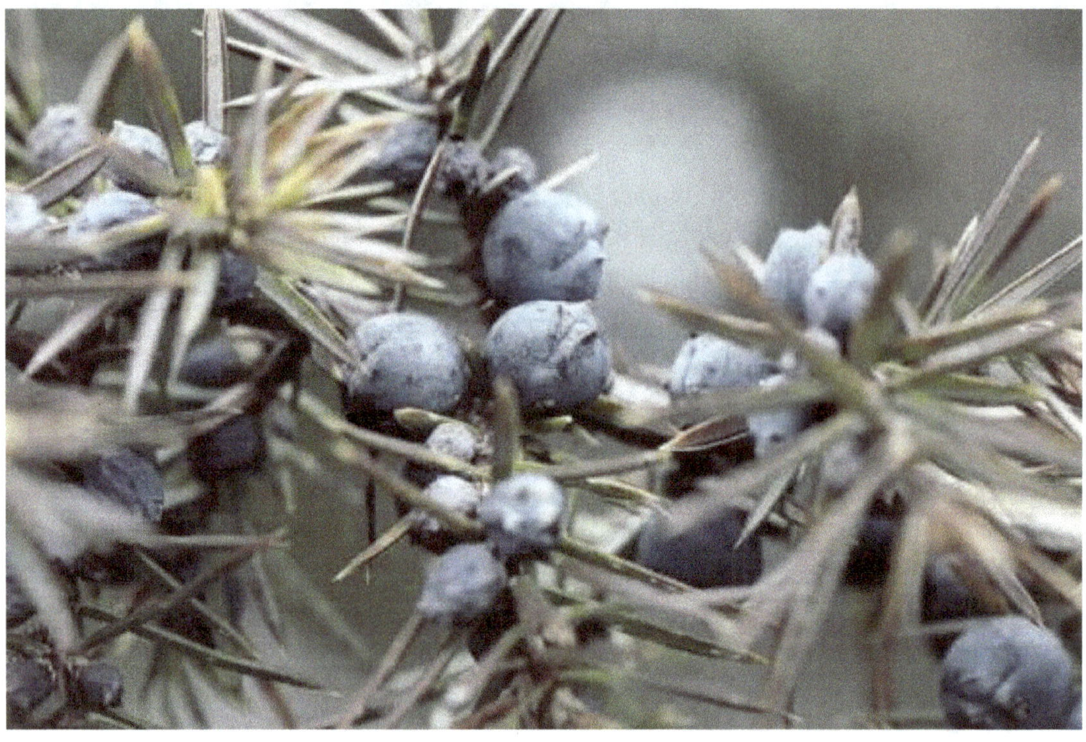

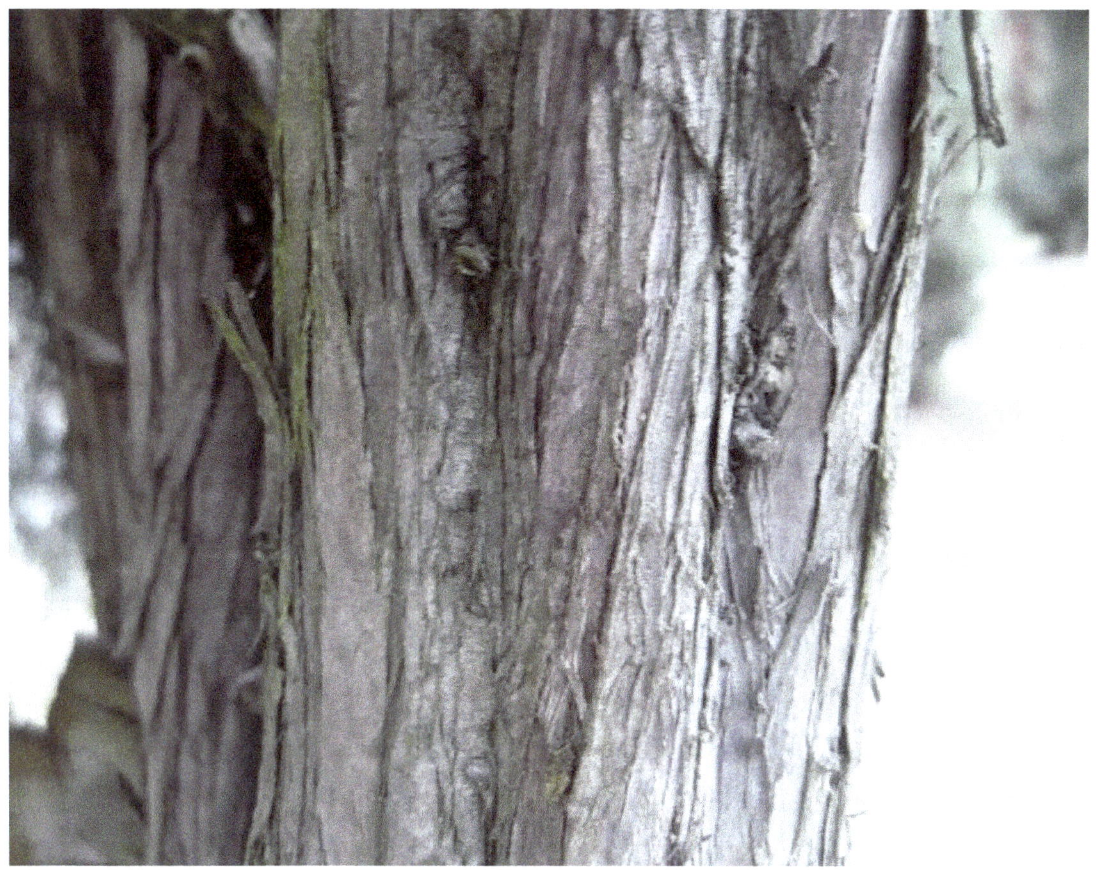

- **Leaves**

Juniper has prickly, evergreen, small, blue-green needles arranged in clusters of three that are rigid and feature a central white stripe.

Its bushiness gives it a minor resemblance to gorse in appearance; however, in contrast to gorse, it exhibits a more sluggish rate of regeneration following fires.

- **Flowers**

Male blossoms are yellow and small in size. Female blossoms emerge between May and June and are green in color.

Flowers of each gender are produced on distinct plants. The breeze is responsible for pollinating the flowers.

- **Fruits**

Juniper fruits resemble berries and are cone-shaped structures composed of succulent scales. When mature, they transform from green in the first year to blue or purple-black in the second. Typically, each fruit contains three rigid, triangular seeds.

- **Bark**

It has a reddish-brown bark. It peels and shreds into segments. Juniper is a long-lived and slow-growing plant. Plants have a maximum lifespan of 2000 years.

- **Flavor**

Clear, fresh and pine-like in flavour, the juniper berries are intensely aromatic when crushed and added to your cooking. The distinctive scent of juniper is immediately reminiscent of gin. It is the only spice that comes from a conifer and is in fact a pine cone with a fleshy covering.

- **Edible parts**

Both leaves and berries

Season

While sowing junipers in the spring is optimal, early autumn can also be a viable alternative.

Habitat

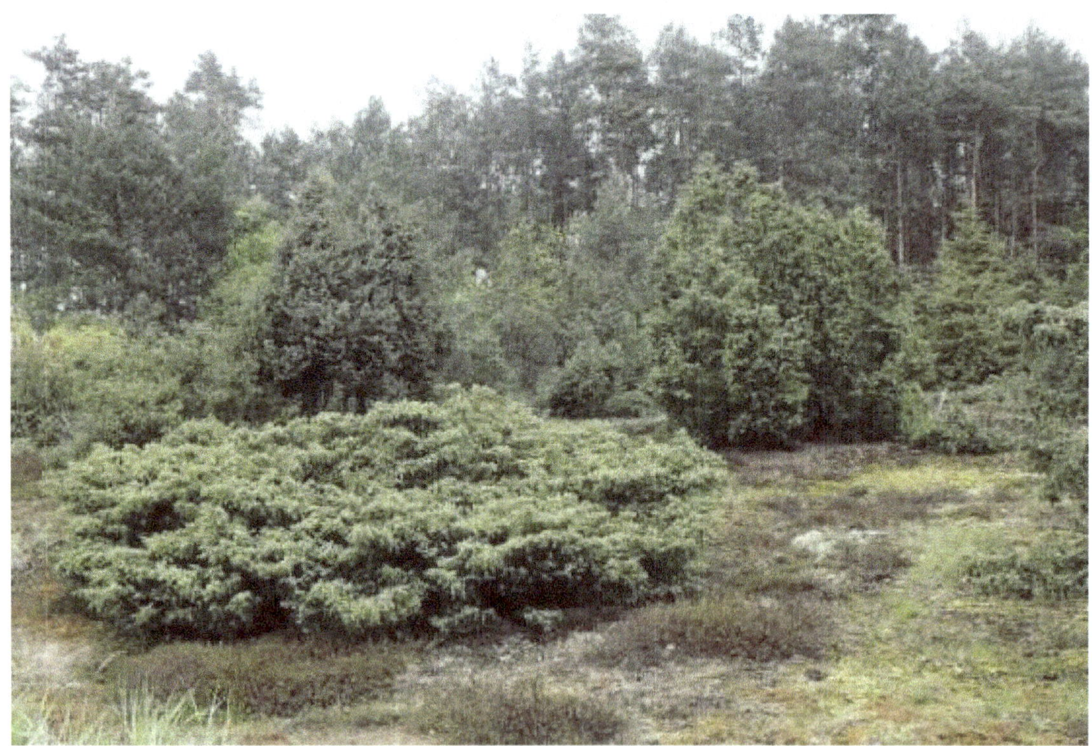

It prefers lime-rich, arid, rocky slopes, chalk downs, heathlands, and moors.

While it exhibits various morphological characteristics, its preferred growth site in Northern Ireland is exposed slopes, where it is typically prostrate (situated near the ground) and seldom exceeds a height of 3 meters. It favors open, sunlit areas and typically produces montane scrub vegetation.

Medicinal Uses

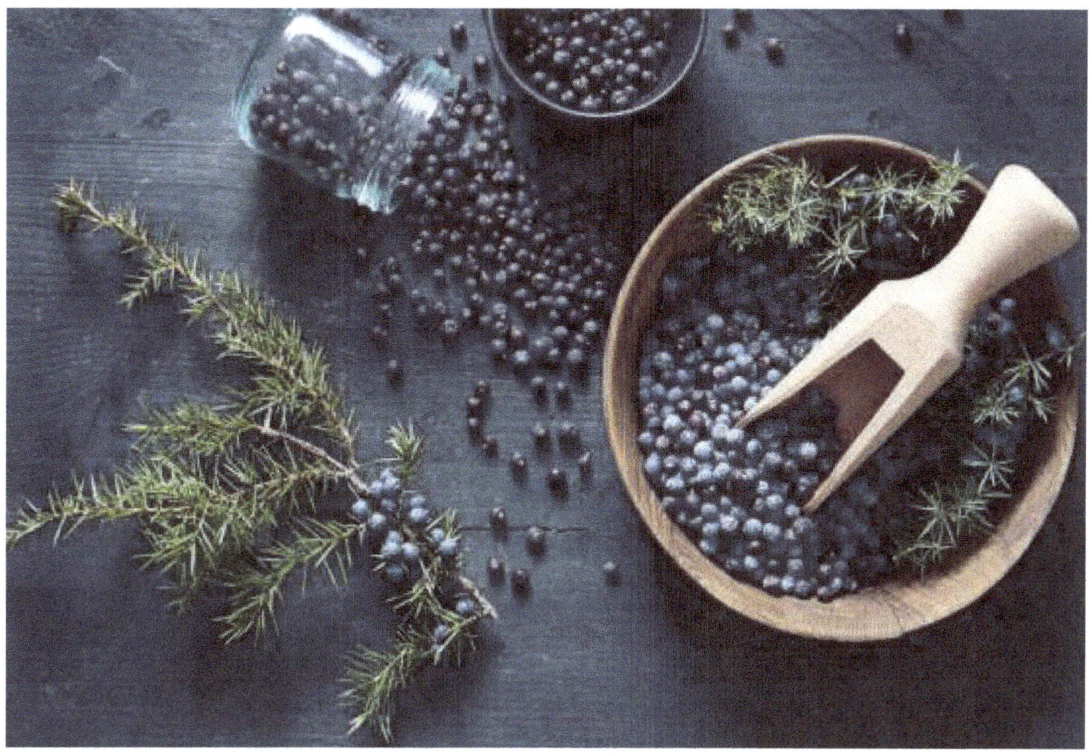

Juniper berries possess numerous potent medicinal properties. As a potent diuretic, juniper is an herb that stimulates the kidneys and aids in the elimination of surplus fluids by increasing urinary output.

This results in the elimination of uric acid and surplus crystals, which are known to induce various complications such as arthritis, kidney stones, and gout.

Terpinen-4-ol, which is abundant in the berries, is a volatile oil that reportedly enhances filtration from the kidneys, thereby increasing urine flow and aiding in the elimination of pathogens from the bladder and kidneys.

As a consequence, Juniper exhibits remarkable efficacy in the management of urinary tract infections; certain users have reported alleviation within a brief span of 24-72 hours. Juniper is even listed in the British Pharmacopoeia as a urinary tract disinfectant.

The potential of the berries to combat liver cancer is presently under investigation owing to their substantial concentration of alpha-pinene compounds.

Additionally, they have been utilized to alleviate uterine issues, toothaches, stomach problems, joint pain, respiratory issues (including asthma), and heart problems (including an irregular pulse).

Furthermore, there is widespread belief that unadulterated juniper berries have the potential to enhance memory function.

Using Juniper for Herbal Purposes

How is juniper utilized medicinally?

Extracts of juniper can be utilized both medicinally and as a dish flavoring. It may be administered topically, inhaled, or ingested as a medication.

The Tanainas in Alaska produce incense by burning juniper needles over a blazing wood fire. In addition to creating a pleasant aroma, this can also help alleviate a chill. Numerous additional juniper herbal applications begin with juniper berry or scale extracts.

A compound known as terpinen-4-ol is present in the preparations; it stimulates the kidneys. They also contain amentoflavone, an additional antiviral compound. Begin by removing juniper needles from your garden shrub if you wish to burn them. It requires little to produce a potent odor.

If one desires alternative herbal applications for juniper beyond combustion, it is possible to procure juniper in commercially available varieties. Consider purchasing oil, tea, and lotion capsules. Occasionally, juniper is consumed in the form of tea. This is reportedly an effective remedy for bronchitis.

It has the potential to alleviate pain, combat inflammation, and stimulate gastric acid production. Additionally, it is purported to cleanse the urinary tract.

Herbal practitioners assert that juniper tea aids in the elimination of superfluous bodily fluids. This diuretic effect eliminates superfluous uric acid from the body. Additionally, due to its high natural insulin content, juniper may lower blood sugar levels.

Additionally, juniper essential oil can be applied topically. When applied topically, it has the potential to alleviate skin conditions such as athlete's foot and acne. Eczema, cystitis, psoriasis, warts, and skin growths are among the conditions that some individuals employ it to treat.

Alongside scaleberry oil, juniper wood can also be utilized to produce an oil. It is known as cade oil and is regarded as a crucial remedy for scalp psoriasis. Due to its antibacterial properties, juniper oil can be applied topically to address skin injuries such as snakebites. Additionally, apply the oil to the skin for relief from joint and muscle discomfort.

Safety Precautions to Be Considered Before Taking Juniper Berries

Juniper berries, when orally consumed in small quantities, are safe, but you still have to be cautious about consuming them.

- It is not advisable for pregnant women to consume juniper berries or juniper berry extracts due to the potential damage they may cause to the unborn child through uterine contraction. Moreover, individuals with kidney conditions should refrain from consuming it due to the potential for renal injury.
- It is not advisable to apply concentrated juniper berry extracts to the skin, as they can induce rashes or, in more severe instances, blister dermatitis

Ingestion of juniper fruit in excess may result in severe adverse effects. Consequently, proceed to the following section to discover the appropriate dosage.

How to Grow

Whatever variety of juniper you decide to cultivate, you must locate a location that meets their specific requirements.

- **Preference location**

Junipers prefer locations that receive either direct sunlight or partial shadow. Although they have no particulars regarding soil type or pH, they dislike wet conditions and require a moist, free-draining soil or growing medium.

A location that is either exposed or sheltered will suffice, and that location need not have an excessive amount of shade as long as it offers nearly every aspect.

Certain junipers are ideal for use as specimen trees that stand alone or as privacy screening plants along the perimeter of a garden.

Others are suitable for the border or the center of a bed.

Low-growing, ground-covering junipers may be utilized as pathway edging or at the front of a plot.

- **Propagation Methods**

Junipers are typically acquired in container form.

However, if you already have juniper in your garden, propagating it through the use of semi-hardwood cuttings in late summer or early autumn is frequently conceivable.

This is the most straightforward method for acquiring new vegetation.

Layering is an additional method of propagation for junipers that is comparatively uncomplicated.

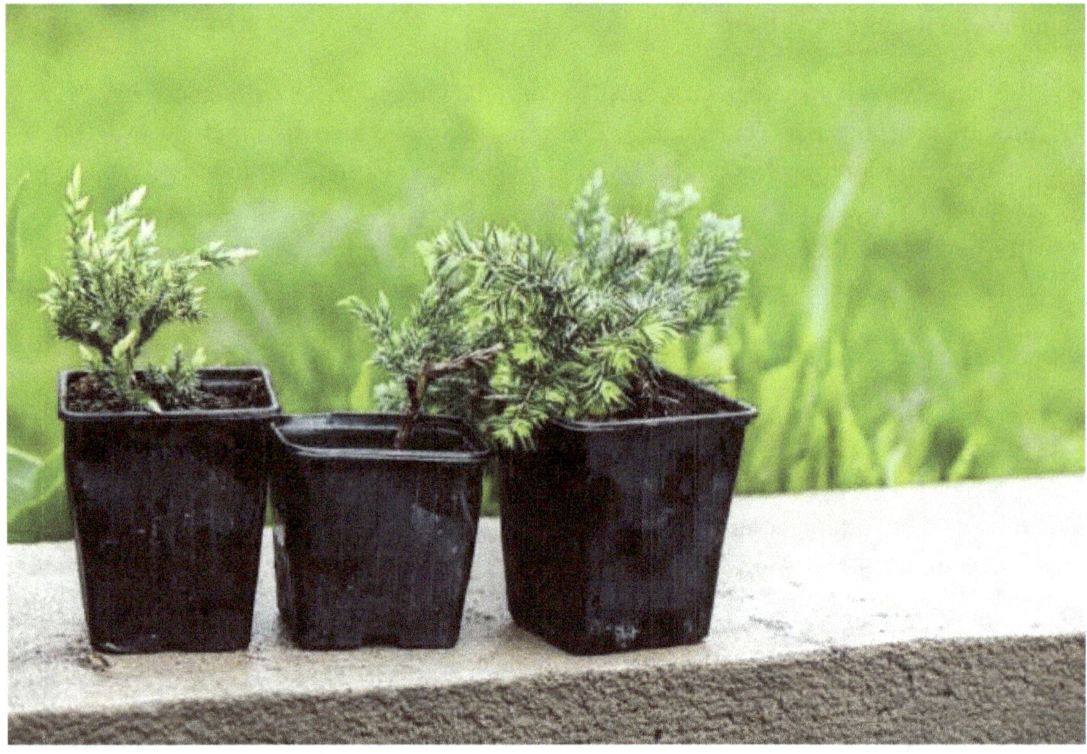

This is accomplished by bending a flexible branch to the ground and maintaining it below the surface of the earth so that it can root.

Nevertheless, this is typically a lengthy procedure, and stratified branches might not germinate for several years.

There is also the possibility that junipers of the same species type can be grown from seed, although this can be a difficult undertaking and the progeny may lack many of the parent plant's characteristics.

Lastly, grafting is another method of propagation utilized with junipers; however, this is a difficult process that home cultivators rarely attempt.

Planting

While junipers thrive in the spring or fall, it is generally possible to plant purchased trees or shrubs outside at virtually any time of year.

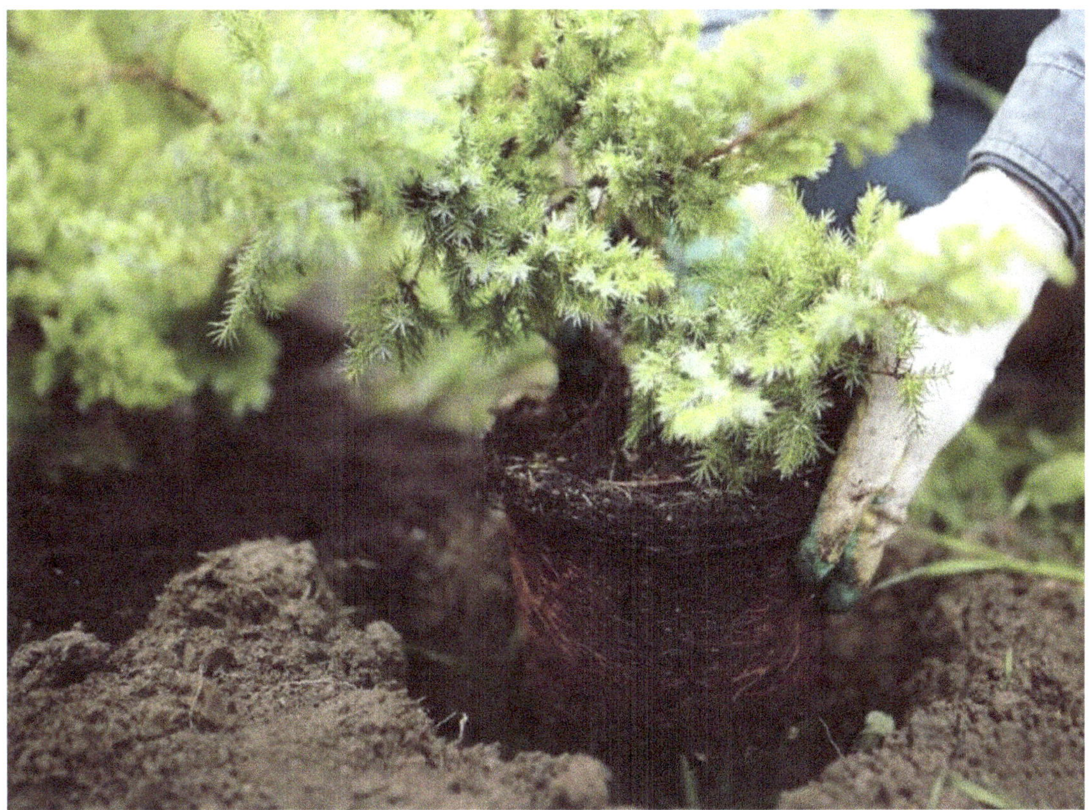

Nevertheless, their establishment may be sluggish in less-than-ideal conditions; therefore, once more, ensure that you select the proper location.

Juniper Care Guidelines

Gaining knowledge about the fundamental requirements of Juniper trees and vegetation can assist in ensuring that they receive the appropriate maintenance.

- **Light Requirements**

Juniper requires either full sun or moderate shade; it cannot thrive in a position that is completely shaded.

In environments with insufficient light, junipers may experience stunted growth and develop into subpar specimens.

- **Soil requirement**

While junipers do not exhibit significant sensitivity towards soil type and pH, it is important to keep in mind that they require moist yet well-draining or free-draining conditions. Waterlogged conditions are intolerable for them.

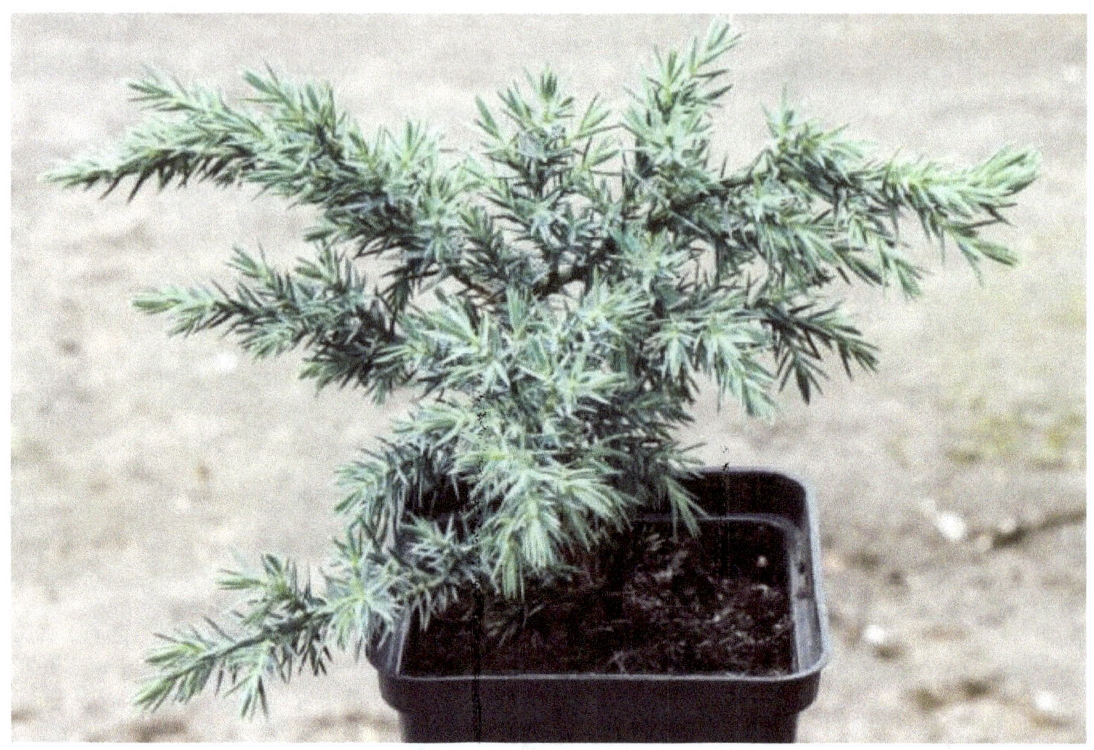

It is essential to maintain adequate drainage, whether cultivating in containers or on the soil.

- **Watering**

Until a juniper becomes established and is grown in containers, water during periods of drought. However, once established, junipers planted in the soil should typically obtain adequate water from rainfall in the Canada.

- **Feeding**

Juniper plants do not exhibit a high level of appetite and typically do not require supplementary nourishment beyond the application of mulch during sowing around the shrub or tree. This mulch should be removed annually in the spring.

Container-grown junipers may occasionally benefit from a weak compost tea or other general-purpose organic liquid fertilizer when growth is inadequate.

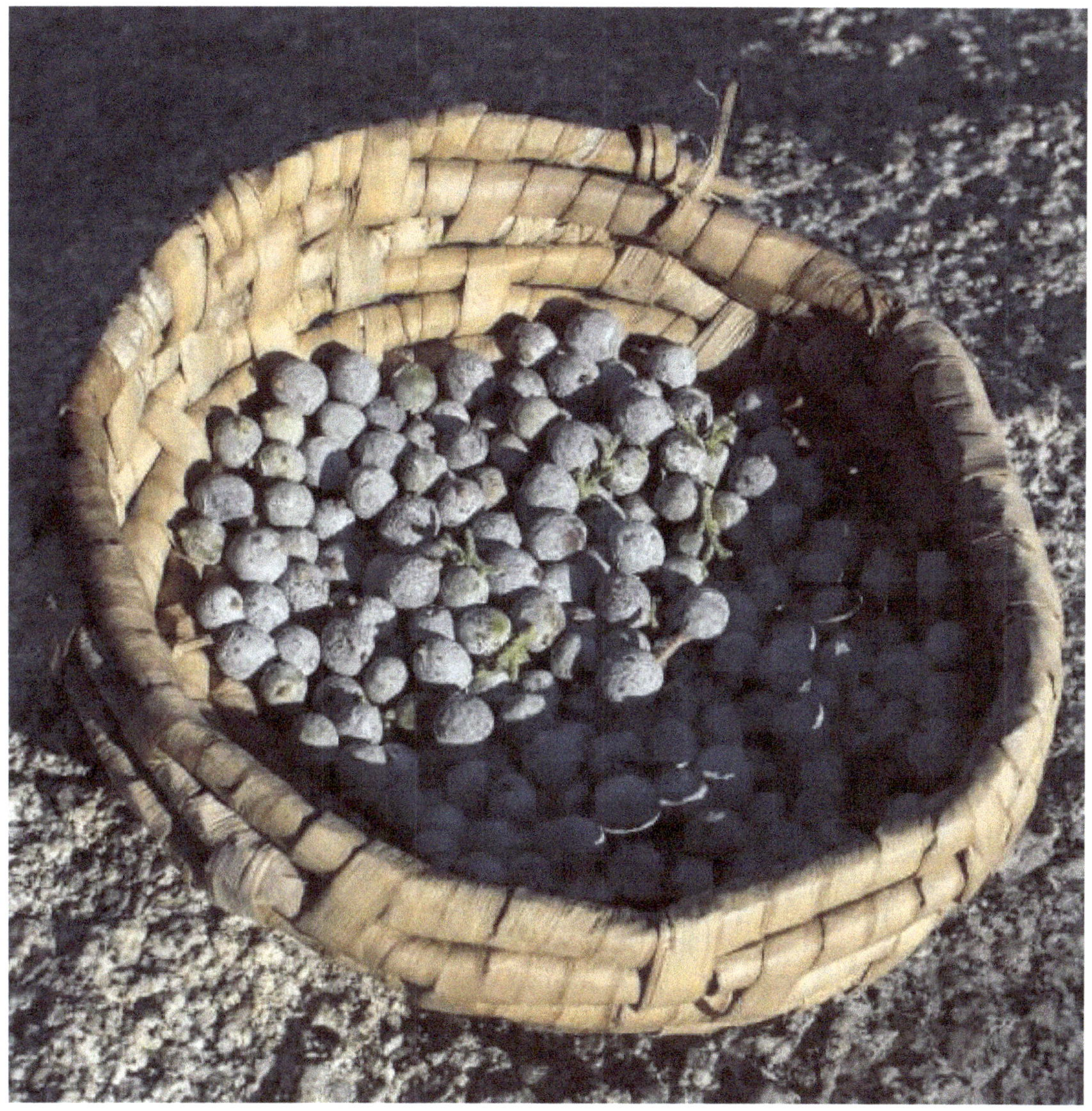

Juniper berries are typically most manageable to harvest during the winter season, when they are mature and have taken on a blue-gray hue. It is imperative to possess prior knowledge of the desired items prior to embarking on a juniper hunt, as with any other foraging endeavor.

When they begin to wrinkle and transform into a dark, purplish-almost-black hue, the berries are mature and ready to be harvested. If they are harvested prematurely, they will lack the desired flavor and become unappealing.

When they reach a deep purple or dark blue hue, they are deemed mature for harvest. The fruit transitions from green to blue before reaching a deep purple hue. Ensure that the juniper berries you harvest are located in regions of the plant that appear to be flourishing.

While winter is the optimal time for me to harvest, depending on where you reside, they can be harvested throughout the year. The blossoms develop from late summer until autumn, when they begin to burst. With the ripening season in mind, the fruit will persist on the bush from early spring to late winter.

Manual picking of juniper fruit is a straightforward undertaking. One may effortlessly remove them from the bush by using their fingertips, although pruning shears may also be employed.

Additionally, I derive pleasure from foraging because it affords me the opportunity to commune with nature while gathering sustenance and medicine.

Dosing

Based on anecdotal evidence, the recommended daily intake of whole or crushed juniper berries is 2–10 grams, whereas juniper berry supplements can be ingested in the range of 1-6 grams.

However, there is a lack of research concerning the precise dosage required to experience the medicinal advantages of these berries.

Furthermore, the optimal dosage is contingent upon factors such as age, health status, and mode of juniper berry ingestion (fresh, dried, extract, or supplement). Before beginning any new supplement, therefore, it is advisable to consult a healthcare professional, as individual responses may differ.

Methods for Drying and Preserving

How is juniper dried?

You may dehydrate the berries overnight in a dehydrator to hasten the drying process, or you may simply let them dry naturally.

Juniper berries are best preserved in an airtight container that is kept in a cold, dry, and dark location. This can aid in the preservation of the berries' flavor and aroma for a period of up to two years by preventing air and moisture damage.

CHAPTER ELEVEN

TURMERIC

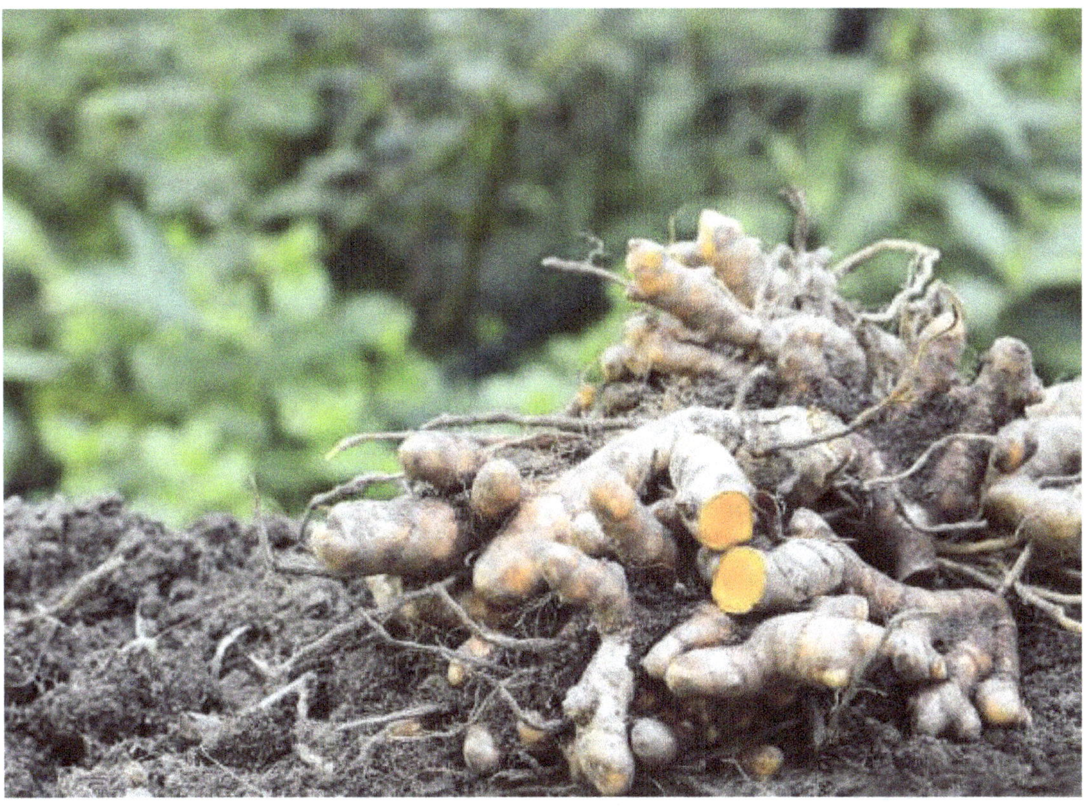

Turmeric (Curcuma longa), an herbaceous member of the ginger family, is the turmeric plant. The exact whereabouts of the plant are unknown; nevertheless, it is hypothesized that it originated in the tropical regions of the Indian Subcontinent or Southeast Asia.

Plentiful precipitation and warm temperatures are required for the plant's development. The plant achieves a vertical height of over three feet, has considerable verdant foliage, and is identified by its sturdy tuberous roots and rhizomes, from which the highly regarded spice is extracted.

The turmeric root, a compound that is widely acknowledged, is employed in the manufacturing process of its distinctive yellow powder.

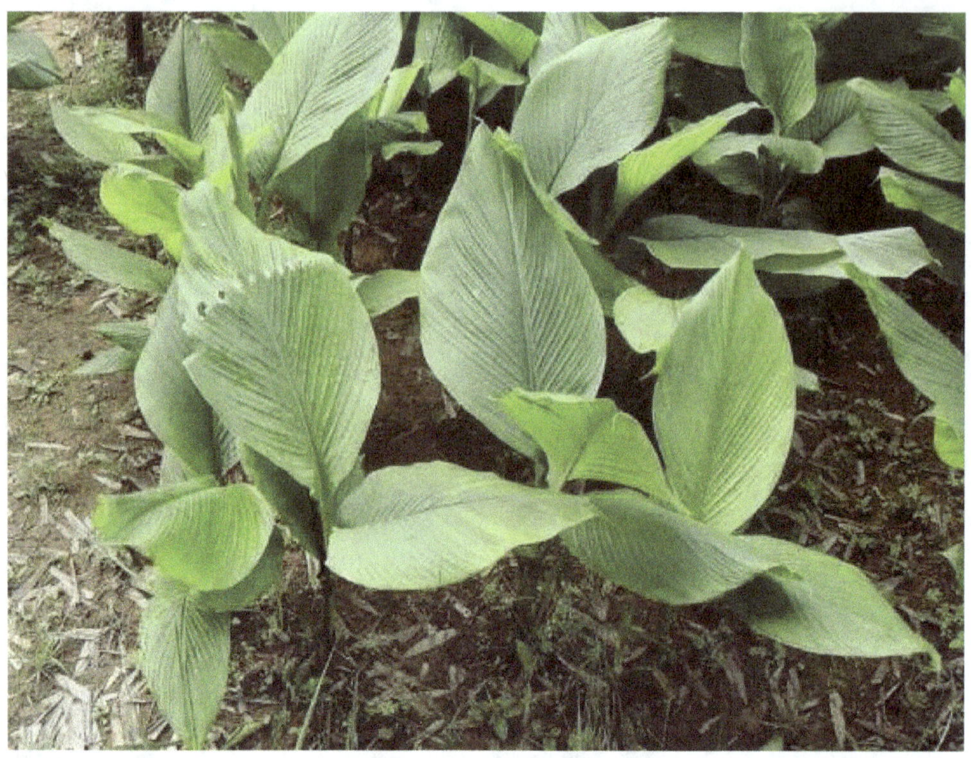

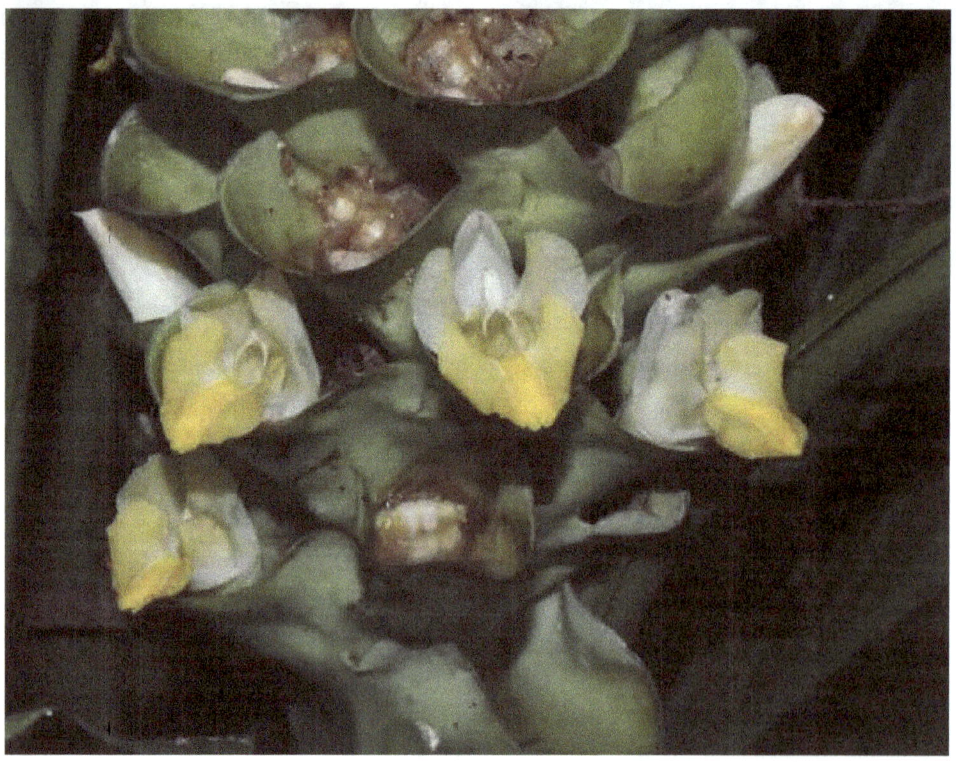

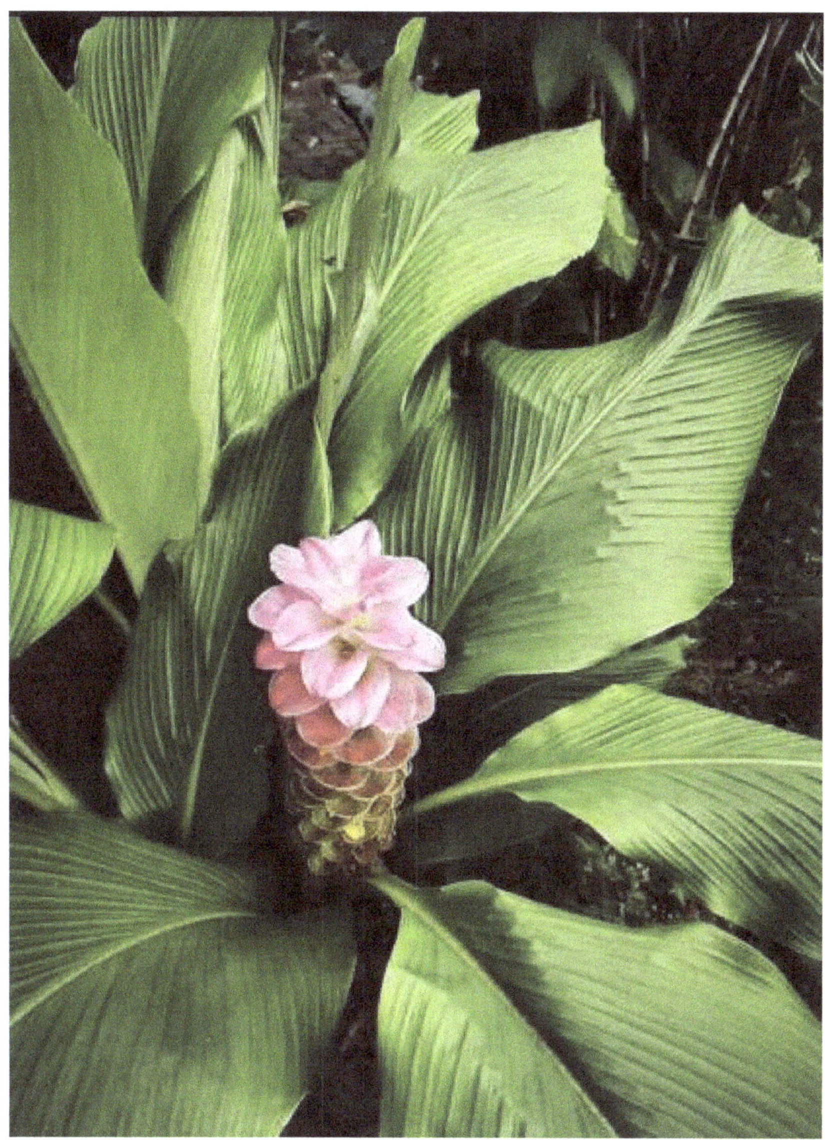

- **Leaves**

Curcumin leaves are elongated, broad, and lance-shaped. They have a maximum length of two feet and are composed of a green hue. A petiole (stalk) that protrudes serves to join the foliage to the stem.

- **Stem**

The slender, underground stem of the turmeric plant produces rhizomes. The rhizomes constitute the primary consumable constituent and are utilized in the production of turmeric spice.

- **Flowers**

Turmeric flowers are relatively small in size, consisting of three petals. Whether they are yellow, white, or pink is contingent upon the variety.

- **Flavor**

Turmeric possesses a warm, bitter, and delicately pungent flavor. Its flavor is earthy, and its aroma is commonly likened to mustard.

- **Edible part**

The primary edible constituent of turmeric is the rhizome, which is extracted for culinary and medicinal purposes. Nevertheless, specific dishes may also integrate the consumable stems and foliage.

Season

Turmeric, being classified as a tropical plant, thrives in balmy and humid conditions. It is customary to fertilize it during the spring and harvest it in the autumn, as the plant requires a duration of seven to ten months to reach maturity.

Habitat

Turmeric plants flourish in well-drained soil and warm, tropical climates. They thrive in environments with temperatures between 68°F and 86°F (20°C and 30°C). In addition to India, China, and Indonesia, numerous tropical regions cultivate turmeric.

Traditional Uses

Thyme has been the focus of considerable scientific inquiry. Anticancer, antimicrobial, anti-inflammatory, and antioxidant properties are all exhibited by it.

It is used in Ayurveda and other traditional medical systems for the treatment of ailments that impact the upper respiratory tract, digestive tract, and epidermis.

Turmeric continues to be utilized traditionally as an herbal remedy. It is purported to provide relief from a range of conditions, including but not limited to allergic reactions, liver disease, digestive disorders, influenza, and arthritis.

According to research, turmeric may have therapeutic advantages for skin health when applied topically or consumed orally. Turmeric has additionally exhibited effectiveness in mitigating joint discomfort associated with arthritis. Participants in one study whose daily intake was 100 milligrams of turmeric extract reported a reduction in joint discomfort.

Ways to Take Turmeric

It's a question we hear a lot!

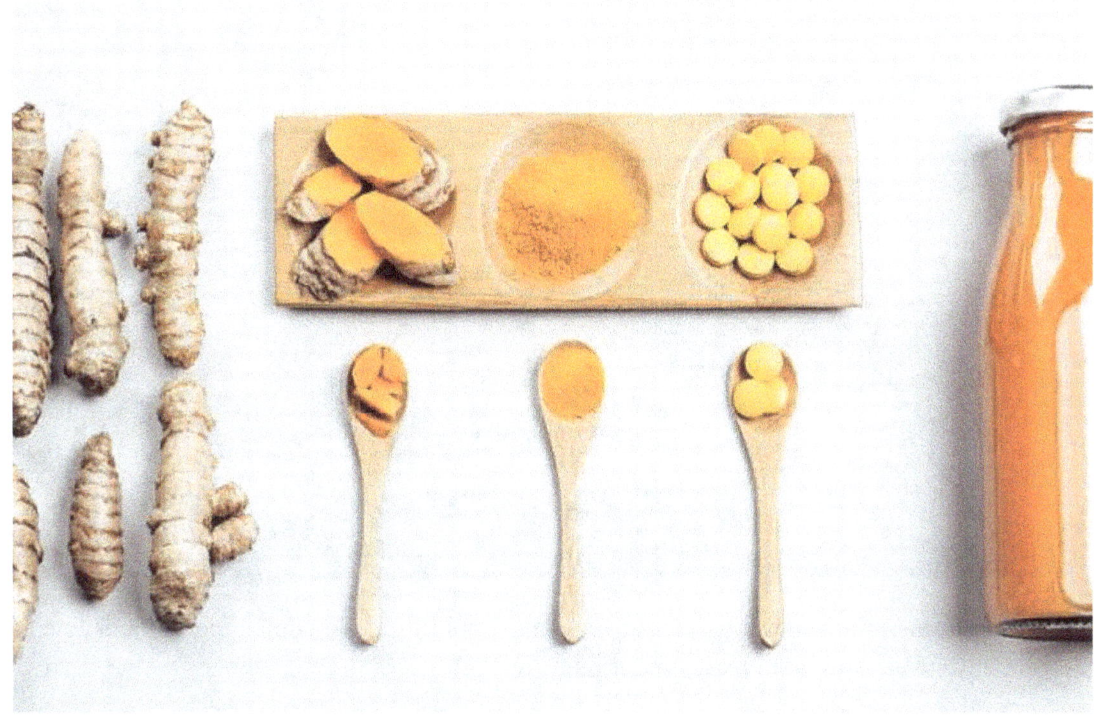

Particularly prevalent in Middle Eastern and South Asian cuisines, turmeric is a fundamental component.

However, as its advantages become more widely known and sought after by experts, its use has expanded to include lattes, popcorn, tablets, and beverages.

However, in order to maximize the body's uptake of the manifold health advantages of turmeric, it is crucial to ascertain the most efficacious mode of administration and determine the optimal dosage of turmeric.

- **Including turmeric in a dish**

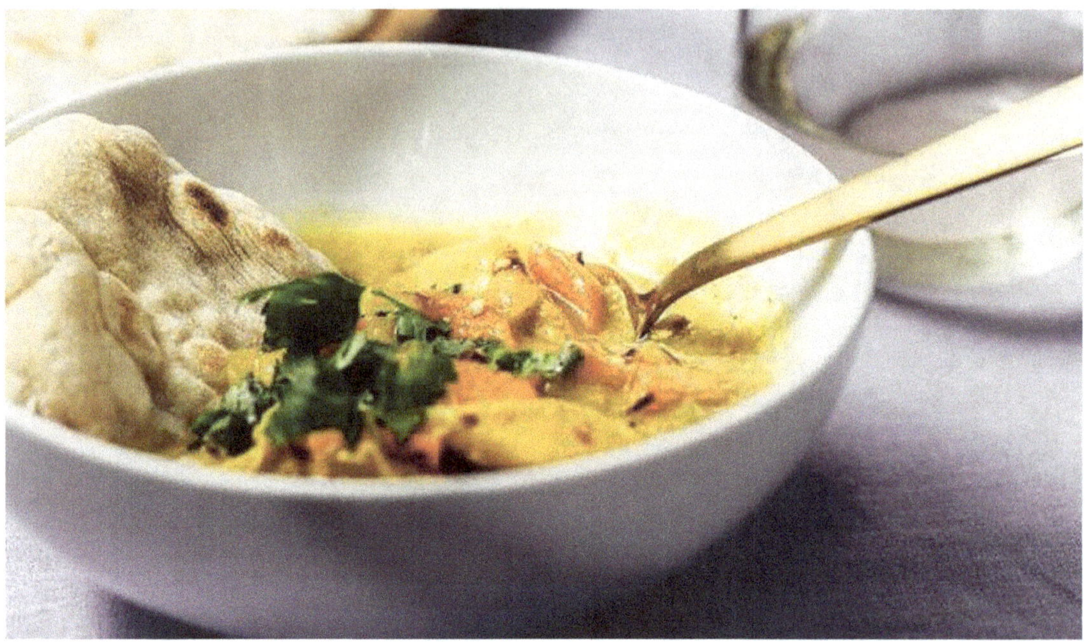

Increasing turmeric intake through the ingestion of more turmeric-containing foods is one of the most common ways to increase turmeric intake.

Curries such as rendang and goan incorporate turmeric into their traditional formulations, whereas recipes for modern foodstuffs, including crackers and popcorn, purposefully call for turmeric as a key ingredient.

An advantageous aspect of integrating turmeric into a dish or beverage is that it offers a practical way to increase one's consumption of turmeric.

This method, particularly for individuals who are unable or reluctant to take turmeric capsules, enables them to augment their daily turmeric consumption without the necessity of doing so.

Nevertheless, is this the most effective approach to consuming turmeric? To state it simply, no. Due to the influence of variables like ingredient usage, portion size, and the ingredient's proportion to the overall meal, accurate regulation of turmeric intake is difficult to achieve.

- **Ingestion of turmeric tablets**

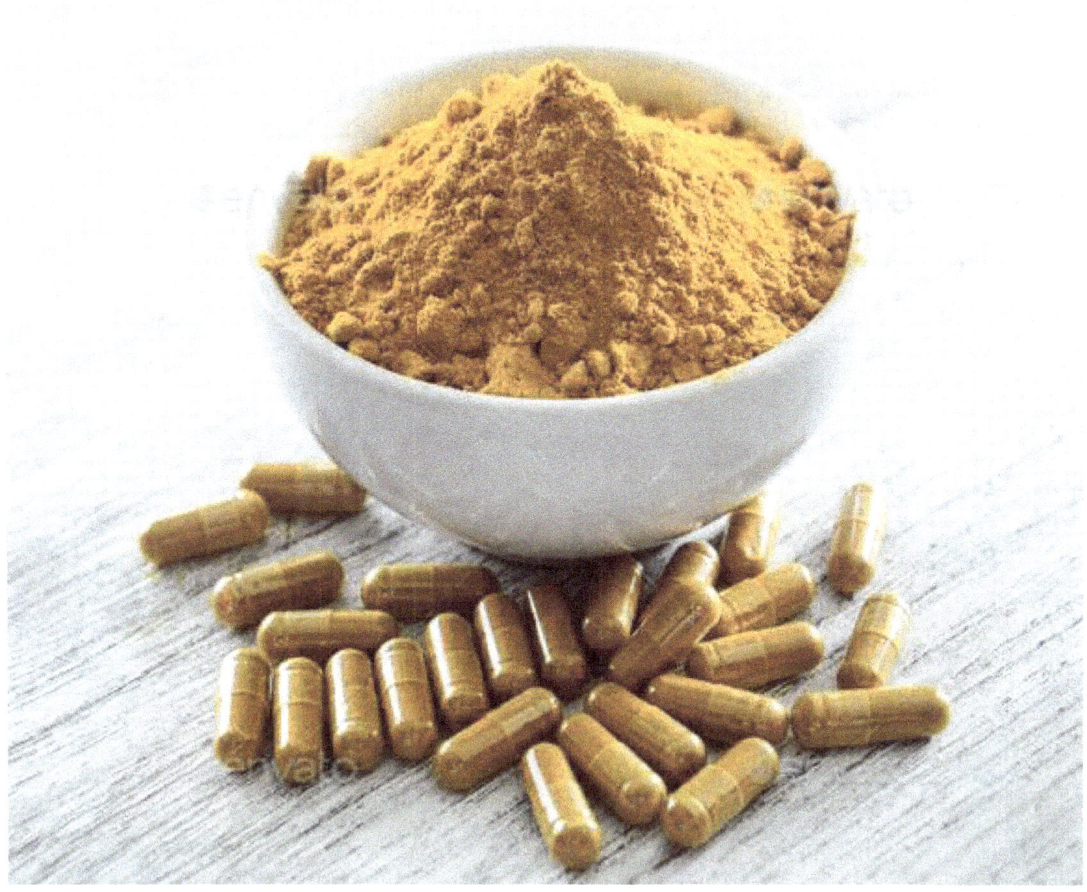

Tablets and capsules containing turmeric are widely available, but their price and ingredient quality can vary significantly. Despite the fact that the abundance of options may make it difficult to find the right tablet, consuming a tablet to increase the amount of turmeric in your diet is a straightforward and simple way to do so, as it provides easy dosage control.

As mentioned earlier, the principal disadvantage of tablets is their solid state, which impedes the body's capacity to absorb the nutrients with the same velocity and efficacy as when they are ingested in liquid form or contained within a liquid capsule!

Why not substitute those tasteless turmeric tablets with a shot of sour, fresh turmeric containing vitamin C and D3? Viva to that!

- **Taking turmeric as a shot**

An effective and palatable approach to consuming a turmeric supplement involves the use of a liquid injection containing a significant quantity of turmeric.

By incorporating turmeric into a premium concoction, one can additionally obtain the advantageous effects of various palatable components. To provide an example, should your turmeric shoot contain ginger, you should consume the following:

- Thiamine is a vital nutrient that facilitates the consistent functioning of the cardiovascular system.
- Riboflavin, an organic compound, facilitates the alleviation of fatigue.
- Vitamin C, which is vital for bone and ligament health maintenance

Both delicious and nutritious!

- **Turmeric added to drinks**

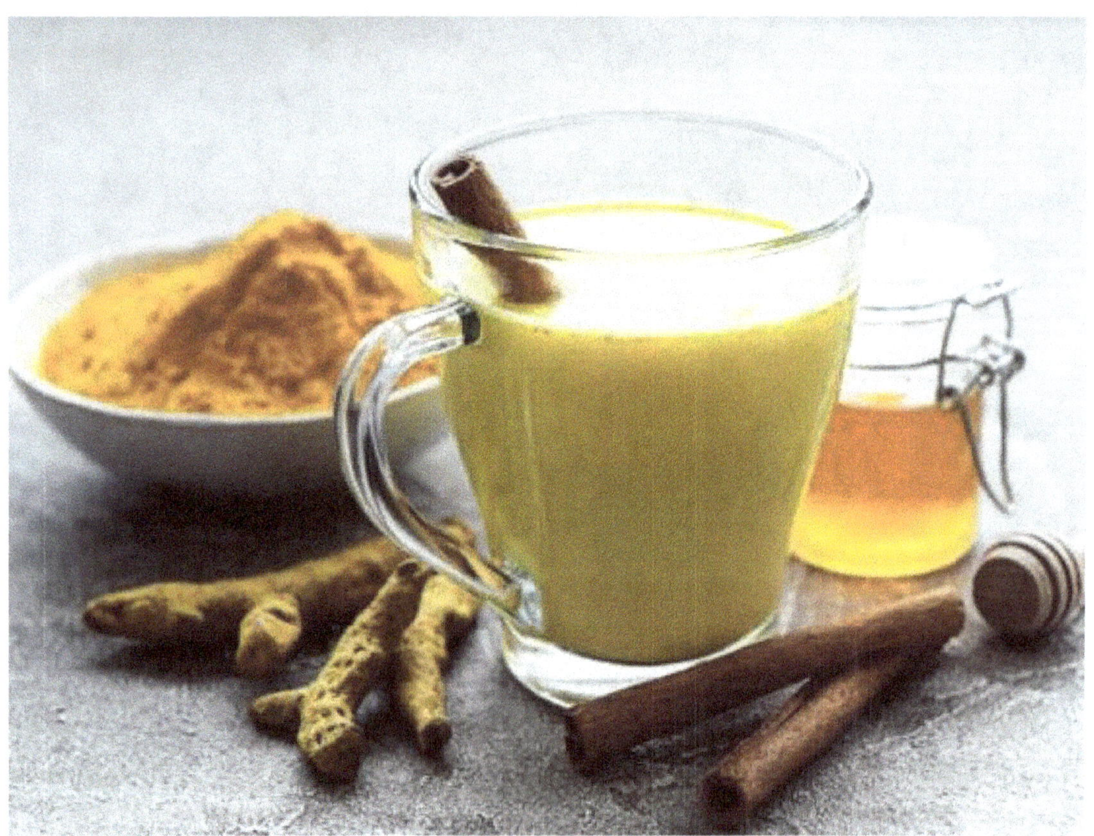

An alternative beneficial approach to consuming turmeric is by means of a beverage, which enhances the probability of efficient nutrient absorption, analogous to the process that would occur with an injection.

The practice of incorporating turmeric into beverages, including lattes, smoothies, and teas, is becoming increasingly prevalent in specialty cafés and restaurants across the nation.

To acquire the prescribed amount of turmeric juice, merely mix one dose into a morning fruit beverage and relish.

- **Curcumin in lubricants**

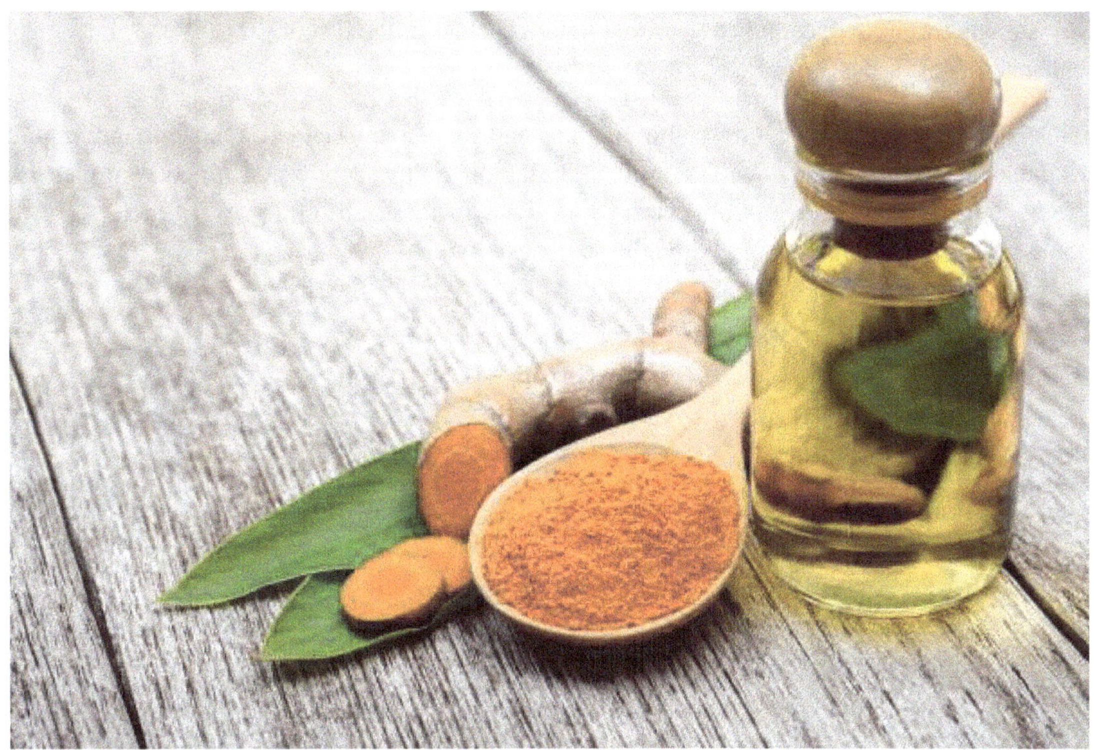

It is worth mentioning that turmeric is additionally detected in essential oils and aromatherapy.

In spite of the paucity of scientific evidence supporting their use as a means of imbibing the benefits of active ingredients, aromatherapy oils will undoubtedly have a potent aroma.

Given that imbibing turmeric via oil is not the most optimal approach, it is exceedingly unlikely that supplementation with turmeric will yield the desired results.

Alternately, if you desire to establish a serene ambiance within your residence, you may combine turmeric oil with fragrances of lemon, nutmeg, and ginger to produce an unparalleled, invigorating scent! Consider combining turmeric oil with jasmine, ylang-ylang, or lavender for a tranquil fragrance.

- **Raw turmeric**

Although consuming raw, fresh turmeric may cause vertigo due to its strong flavor and viscosity, it provides the ability to precisely control one's intake.

One may partake in the consumption of pure turmeric in numerous forms, including powdered or grated varieties. To maximize absorption and enhance palatability, it is recommended to incorporate turmeric into a liquid medium, such as a smoothie, flavored turmeric shot, or turmeric tea.

The best way to take turmeric

Consuming turmeric in conjunction with a liquid, such as a liquid shot, smoothie, or beverage, enhances its efficacy.

This is because the body requires solid vitamins and supplements (such as those found in food or tablets) to be broken down prior to assimilation of the active constituents' properties. Combining turmeric and ground black pepper can increase absorption by a factor of two thousand. Doubts cannot be placed on the statistics!

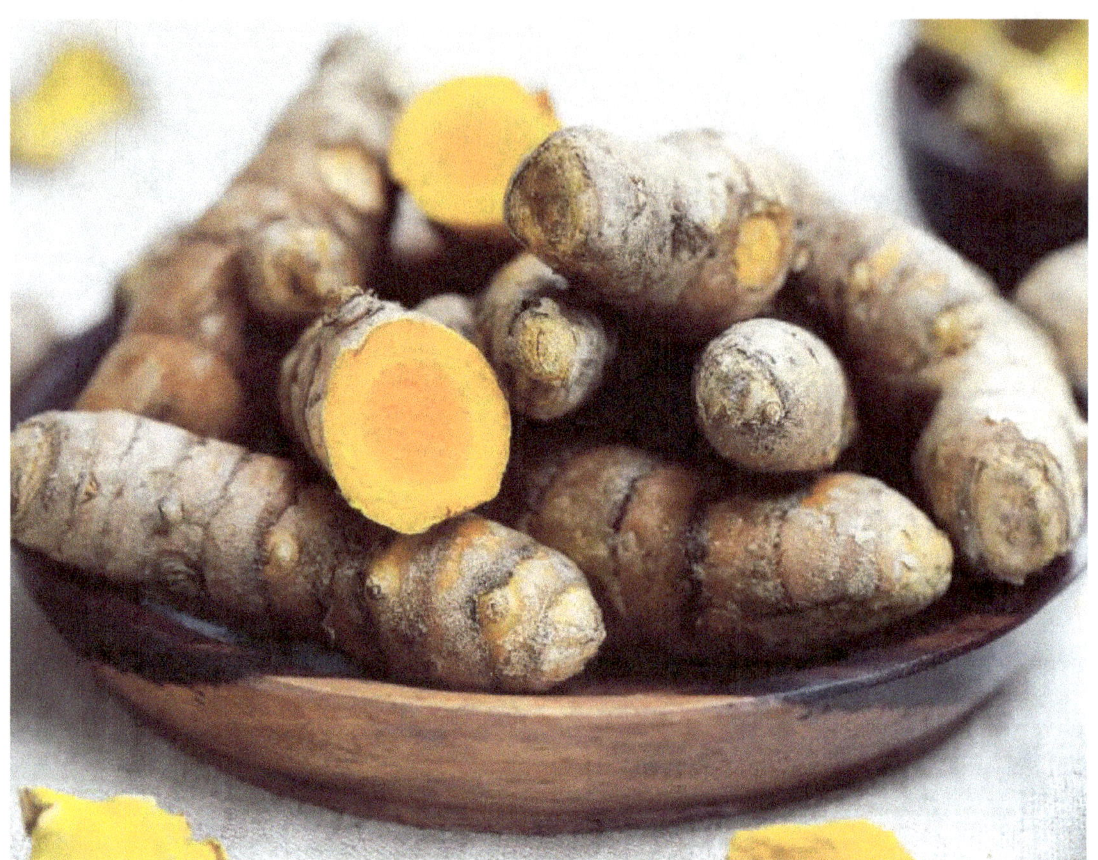

How to Grow

Choosing rhizomes is the initial stage in the investigation of turmeric. Conduct an internet search or visit a horticultural center in search of fresh, healthy turmeric rhizomes. Each portion should be substantial, consisting of at least two to three blossoms.

- **Preparing Your Rhizomes**

Rhizome preparation should occur prior to sowing. When feasible, partition larger rhizomes into smaller segments, taking care to restrict the number of blossoms in each segment. These items can be kept dry for one to two days to avert decay and illness.

- **Selecting the ideal location**

The optimal location for sowing must then be identified. Turmeric plants flourish in temperate climates characterized by sufficient humidity and sunlight. Nevertheless, they are tolerant of some shade. One need not be concerned if they happen to reside in a frigid region. Indoor cultivation of this plant is feasible in the vicinity of a window that receives natural light or beneath grow lighting.

- **Prepare the soil.**

Soil that drains adequately is essential for the cultivation of turmeric. To enhance drainage, it is possible to integrate compost, silt, or perlite into the ideal composition. Soil pH should ideally fall within the range of 6.0 to 7.0, which corresponds to a modestly acidic to neutral state.

- **Plant your turmeric.**

You are now permitted to begin sowing. The turmeric rhizomes that have been prepared should be inserted into the soil at a depth of approximately two inches, with the blossoms facing upward. When planting multiple rhizomes, allow 12 to 16 inches of space between each one to facilitate growth. The soil should be thoroughly moistened before sowing.

How to Take Care of a Turmeric Plant

Turmeric requires ongoing maintenance following its initial sowing to ensure its optimal growth. Bear in mind the subsequent maintenance requirements

- **Watering**

Excessive irrigation is critical to prevent rot, despite the fact that turmeric can thrive in saturated soil. While it is generally recommended to irrigate vegetation every two days, this schedule can be modified to accommodate the specific climatic and environmental conditions of the area.

- **Sunlight**

It is imperative that your turmeric plant receive sufficient light. Ensure that it is exposed to light for a minimum of five to six hours daily, either through window exposure or under a grow light, when cultivating it indoors.

- **Fertilizer**

Assist your plant by applying an organic fertilizer that is abundant in nitrogen. Monthly treatments should be administered to ensure that turmeric receives the necessary nutrients to thrive throughout the growth season.

- **Exert patience as the turmeric plant develops.**

Tremendous patience is required for the cultivation of turmeric. Several months may pass before seedlings begin to emerge from the soil. In the absence of any imminent occurrences, there is no reason to be concerned. At this moment, your plant is actively involved in the development of considerable subterranean roots.

Harvesting

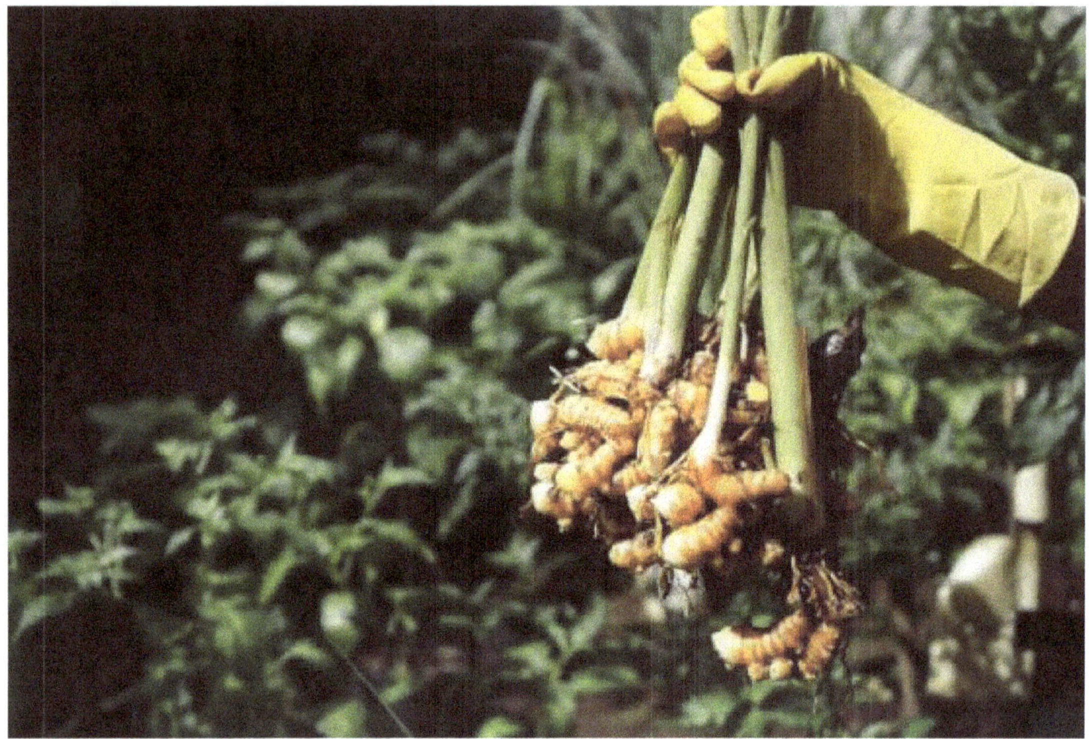

In autumn, when the foliage begins to wilt and expire, it is prudent to pick up the plants with care.

Gradually extract complete plants from the soil by circling them with a garden fork while simultaneously applying downward pressure with your foot and flexing the fork in a bending motion.

At the apex, where the foliage meets the roots, eliminate and dispose of the foliage. Fresh turmeric is harvested from the "hands" of the remaining rhizomes.

Dosing

Research has demonstrated that curcumin, in doses as high as 2,000 mg, is harmless for human consumption and aids in the functioning of bodily systems.

Our core range shots consist of 35 grams of unprocessed turmeric rhizome, which is abundant in curcumin. To avoid an elaborate mathematical explanation, this means that an approximate amount of 1,750 mg of curcumin is present in each injection, along with a multitude of other components and compounds!

Preserving

Frozen raw tubers are stored in a hermetic zippered plastic bag after being stored in a mesh bag for refrigeration. Slicing or grating them as required

It is possible to store whole rhizomes in refrigeration for a maximum of three months and to freeze them for a duration of six months when cut. Preserve a portion for subsequent seeding seasons.

In addition, the roots can be reduced to a fine powder by drying and boiling them. Wear food-safe mitts and work on a non-stainable surface to prevent the epidermis and counter from turning yellow.

CONCLUSION

As we approach the concluding sections of the manual on edible and medicinal plants of the Rockies, we stand at a juncture where understanding and admiration for the extraordinary vegetation that adorns this alpine region converge. By delving into alpine meadows, dense forests, and winding valleys, we have discovered the concealed treasures that have provided sustenance for generations of both fauna and human beings.

Throughout our expedition, we have beenholden to the tenacity of the natural world and its capacity to not only supply nourishment but also therapeutic attributes intricately woven into the terrain itself. The Rocky Mountains, characterized by their majestic summits and babbling rivers, have evolved into more than a picturesque backdrop; they have also become a veritable pharmacy and a gastronomic paradise awaiting discovery.

We urge you, as you conclude this book, to apply the insights and knowledge acquired from its pages beyond the confines of your reading nook and into the untamed. Explore the Rockies with an enhanced recognition of the precarious equilibrium that exists between fauna and civilization. It is imperative to accept the duty of conscientiously foraging, recognizing the interdependence of all organisms and the significance of safeguarding these botanical marvels for posterity.

May the knowledge and understanding imparted here ignite a more profound affinity for the Earth, cultivating a responsibility to protect the fragile ecosystems that render the Rocky Mountains a sanctuary for an array of flora. This guide ought to inspire and motivate individuals to engage in contemplative exploration, sustainable foraging, and a reverence for the abundant natural resources that encompass us.

Bear in mind, in the pursuit of exploration and preservation, that our connection with the natural world is mutual. In the same way that the vegetation of the Rocky Mountains has provided us with nourishment and therapeutic benefits, it is incumbent upon us to bestow in return an attitude of appreciation, comprehension, and a steadfast dedication to safeguarding the intricate equilibrium that sustains the life of this ecosystem.

Therefore, as one ventures into the rugged wilderness of the Rocky Mountains, may they bear the knowledge acquired here, exercise caution, and discover satisfaction in the symbiotic interaction between sentient beings and the unspoiled splendor of this extraordinary terrain.

"Harvesting Nature's Bounty" serves as more than a mere guide; it extends an invitation to initiate an enduring exploration, reverence, and wonderment for the palatable and therapeutic plants that adorn the magnificent Rocky Mountains.